Hospital Pharmacy Practice for
Technicians

Mark G. Brunton, CPhT

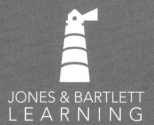

JONES & BARTLETT
LEARNING

World Headquarters
Jones & Bartlett Learning
5 Wall Street
Burlington, MA 01803
978-443-5000
info@jblearning.com
www.jblearning.com

Jones & Bartlett Learning books and products are available through most bookstores and online booksellers. To contact Jones & Bartlett Learning directly, call 800-832-0034, fax 978-443-8000, or visit our website, www.jblearning.com.

Substantial discounts on bulk quantities of Jones & Bartlett Learning publications are available to corporations, professional associations, and other qualified organizations. For details and specific discount information, contact the special sales department at Jones & Bartlett Learning via the above contact information or send an email to specialsales@jblearning.com.

Production Credits

Executive Publisher: William Brottmiller
Executive Editor: Rhonda Dearborn
Senior Managing Editor: Maro Gartside
Editorial Assistant: Sean Fabery
Production Editor: Amanda Clerkin
Marketing Manager: Grace Richards
VP, Manufacturing and Inventory Control: Therese Connell

Composition: Aptara®, Inc.
Cover Design: Michael O'Donnell
Photo Research and Permissions Coordinator: Amy Rathburn
Cover Image: © ULKASTUDIO/ShutterStock, Inc.
Printing and Binding: Edwards Brothers Malloy
Cover Printing: Edwards Brothers Malloy

Library of Congress Cataloging-in-Publication Data

Brunton, Mark G., author.
  Hospital pharmacy practice for technicians/by Mark G. Brunton.
    p.;cm.
  Includes bibliographical references and index.
  ISBN 978-1-284-03046-4—ISBN 1-284-03046-6
  I. Title.
  [DNLM: 1. Pharmacists' Aides—standards.   2. Pharmacy Service, Hospital—standards.
3. Clinical Competence.   4. Clinical Pharmacy Information Systems.   5. Professional Role. QV 21.5]
  RS122.95
  615.1—dc23
                                                                          2013021513

6048

Printed in the United States of America
17 16 15 14 13   10 9 8 7 6 5 4 3 2 1

Dedication

In memory of Charles Alexander Brunton III.
"To everything there is a season, and a time
to every purpose under heaven."
—Ecclesiastes 3:1

Contents

Preface

When teaching pharmacy technician students in the classroom, one of the most frequently asked questions is about the difference between health system and retail pharmacy. In the beginning, my answers would cover some of the major points of divergence. "Health system technicians don't handle insurance billing." "Retail technicians don't compound IVs." "Retail technicians deal directly with patients; health system technicians deal with nurses." And so on and so on. I have come to realize that there are not just minor differences in a few key areas. The very nature of everything is different. Health system pharmacy is a completely different animal in terms of processes, interactions, and workflow.

This text was written for the purpose of giving a student an overview of all aspects of health system pharmacy, not just those "minor areas." By presenting a broad picture of the different duties, technology, and policies of this field, a student will be better prepared to excel in this setting. This falls in line with the standards of accreditation for the American Society of Health-System Pharmacists (ASHP) nicely, because nonretail experiential training is a requirement. By teaching students the proverbial ins and outs of health system practice, their performance will improve when participating in these externships. This will hopefully also increase health system pharmacy's willingness to train students across the board. In addition, this text has a strong professionalism component built in and customized to interactions with health system employees and situations. These chapters are at the front of the text on purpose, with the theory that these skills will prepare a student for improved performance not only in the field, but also in the classroom.

Although the roles and responsibilities of pharmacy technicians are constantly evolving, and technology is growing ever more advanced, the principles in this text will allow a student to hit the ground running and be able to more easily evolve and thrive in this dynamic profession.

About the Author

Mark G. Brunton has served in the field for 10 years as a health system pharmacy technician, and has instructed technician students for 8 years. Mr. Brunton has been a speaker at the American Society for Health-System Pharmacists (ASHP) Midyear Clinical Meeting for 3 years and has served as their Technician Education Committee Chair. He has also been a subject matter expert for the development of a blended curriculum for Kaplan College's pharmacy technician program. Mr. Brunton has also served as the technician representative for the Nevada Society of Health-System Pharmacists (NVSHP), and was awarded Technician of the Year for 2011 by NVSHP. Mr. Brunton was selected to be a panel member for the U.S. Department of Education's National Assessment on Educational Progress conference for vocational training. He is currently a member of the Technician Advisory Committee to the Nevada State Board of Pharmacy. It is his express pleasure to be able to help train a workforce of confident and competent technicians for future practice.

Acknowledgments

I would like to thank the following people for contributing to the inspiration, knowledge, and sanity that went into the creation of this text:

Tari Broderick, for seeing the potential in me as an author. I had not seriously considered the possibility until you walked up to me and floored me with an unbelievable opportunity. Thank you for starting me on this path, and for having such enthusiasm for this text. I owe you a 3C's, and so much more! (Or is it Seas?)

All of my pharmacy students both past and present for asking those questions that dug to the root of that all-pervasive question, "Why?" It is through the delivering of material to you that I have anecdotes and real-life stories to put in this text for many more technicians to learn from.

Valerie Wright, for inspiring me more than I think you realize. I credit you with much of my development as a pharmacy technician, and also as the motivator to go into teaching. Thank you for believing in me.

Nick Barkley, for all of the last minute questions and photo ops. I am truly glad to see how far you have come my friend—no more papers in the Honda Civic!

Liz Martinez, for your insight and confidence boosting. Your advice and critiques got me over some major humps during this process. I owe you that steak dinner.

The editors at Jones & Bartlett Learning, for all of your expertise and help in getting this text published. Sean, Katey, and Teresa, you have been fantastic to work with, thank you so much.

Introduction

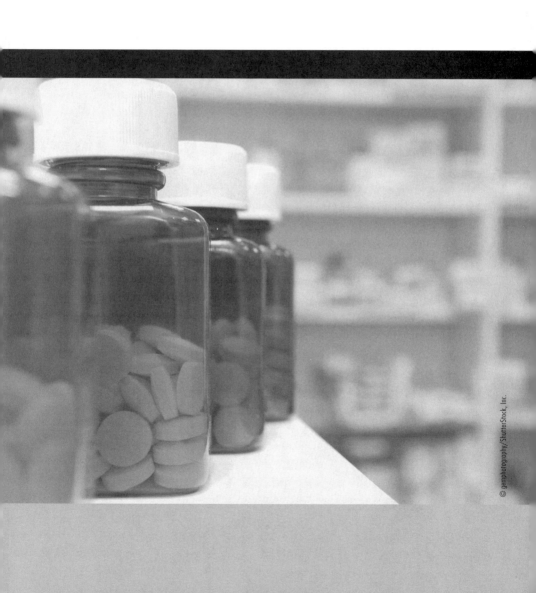

CHAPTER 1

Health System and Pharmacy Technician Overview

LEARNING OBJECTIVES

Upon completion of this chapter, you will be able to

1. Describe the origins of health system pharmacy technicians
2. Understand how the roles and duties of pharmacy technicians have expanded to the present day
3. Comprehend the potential future roles and responsibilities of pharmacy technicians
4. List different departments and care units common in health system settings

KEY TERM

Health system

INTRODUCTION

History is an excellent teacher. To see what has come before and why it has occurred enables one to move forward with greater insight and motivation in any discipline, including in the role of pharmacy technician. This chapter explains the beginnings of the pharmacy technician profession in the health system setting, how the profession has grown in scope, and how it will continue to evolve in the future. By understanding the history and nature of the institutions that shape the field, pharmacy technicians can be more effective, confident, and successful in their positions. We will examine three areas to provide a broader picture of the profession: its beginnings, its evolution and present day incarnation, and its potential future scope. The pivotal factors that have had a large influence on these periods are World War II, the evolution of pharmacist duties, contemporary initiatives, and technologies that are setting the stage for future practice.

ORIGIN OF THE PHARMACY TECHNICIAN

There is no clear date or single event that can be cited for the creation of the pharmacy technician position. Many factors played a part in its inception. Pri-

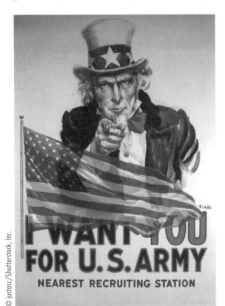

© justasc/Shutterstock, Inc.

FIGURE 1-1 The famous Uncle Sam recruitment poster used during World War II.

or to the designation or title of *pharmacy technician*, there were pharmacy assistants, clerks, or aides. Their roles predominately dealt with the filing of paperwork and other types of clerical duties. These positions evolved into that of a pharmacy technician. Of the many factors that influenced its creation, one of the largest was the beginning and end of World War II. World War II pulled many able-bodied men to the front lines, including pharmacists (**Figures 1-1** and **1-2**). As a result, there was a shortage of pharmacists on the home front, which required aides and clerks to step in and perform more duties to help make up for the deficiency (Worthen, 2004). Also, in the armed services, a pharmacist assistant was a designated

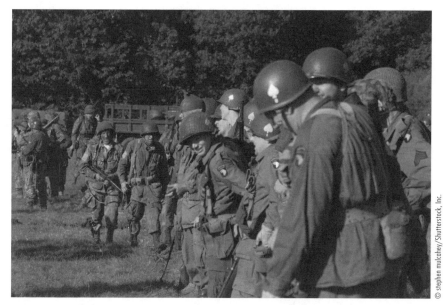

FIGURE 1-2 Many pharmacists joined the armed services during World War II.

position and rank, with dispensing duties and assistance to the pharmacist being the primary role. At the conclusion of hostilities, many of these pharmacist assistants came back to the United States and found employment in hospital pharmacies with roles and duties in the civilian sector comparable to those they performed in the military.

EVOLUTION OF THE PHARMACY TECHNICIAN

As the profession of pharmacy grew over the decades following World War II, the focus of duties in pharmacist training programs and patient care shifted. The primary role of pharmacists prior to the 1970s was mainly *dispensing* medications as prescribed by a physician. This is no doubt where the stereotype of "pill counter" or the nickname of "pill pusher" came into being, because it was the most common activity of pharmacists at that time. As the number of different medications being produced increased, the number of options for medication therapy grew exponentially larger. As a result, pharmacist roles became more centered on medication therapy, as opposed to dispensing. Pharmacists became more involved with activities such as checking drug interactions and contraindications, selection of therapy, and

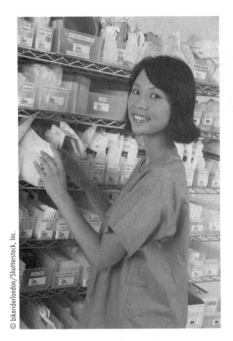

© bikeriderlondon/Shutterstock, Inc.

FIGURE 1-3 A pharmacy technician in a health system setting.

patient care outcomes. These functions centered more on utilizing the pharmacist's clinical knowledge and training. As a result, medication dispensing activities fell more heavily on the pharmacy technician. It was soon recognized that technicians could handle almost all aspects of the preparation of medications, with a pharmacist verifying the work before delivery to the nursing units in a health system setting. This practice set the stage for today's structure of a health system pharmacy.

CURRENT ROLE OF THE PHARMACY TECHNICIAN

At present, pharmacy technicians perform numerous duties in a health system pharmacy's operations (**Figure 1-3**). All of them have one primary goal—dispensing medications to the patient.

The use of technology to dispense medications is a large factor in health system pharmacy. Today's technicians constantly work with various software, hardware, and mechanical devices to increase not only efficiency, but also safety in terms of medication delivery. Technicians are also increasingly assisting the pharmacist with duties relating to medication therapy management.

FUTURE OF THE PHARMACY TECHNICIAN

With the current model of pharmacy practice, the roles, responsibilities, and training of pharmacy technicians are evolving. Professional organizations are promoting higher standards of education and certification. Technicians are also undertaking additional duties in the health system setting. As a result, pharmacists have more time to conduct their clinical duties.

In 2003, the leading national organizations of pharmacy practice endorsed a document published by the American Society of Health-System Pharmacists

(ASHP) known as the "White Paper on Pharmacy Technicians." This document describes the increasing roles of pharmacy technicians. It also recommends standards of training and certification to meet these expanding responsibilities (American Society of Health-System Pharmacists, 2003).

In 2011, the Pharmacy Technician Certification Board (PTCB) held a summit called C.R.E.S.T., composed of leaders in the field of pharmacy. PTCB is the foremost leader in the area of technician certification. The attendees at this summit included pharmacists, technicians, and educators. The summit addressed issues and solicited feedback about future roles and responsibilities for technicians. As a result of this meeting, several initiatives are moving forward for requirements and standards for national certification of technicians. For example, criminal background checks, as well as graduation from an accredited training program, will be necessary before being able to sit for PTCB's national exam. These types of standards will help promote advancement within the profession, and increase the quality of technicians on the whole (C.R.E.S.T. Initiative, 2013).

HEALTH SYSTEM OVERVIEW

A health system is today's term for what has traditionally been known as a hospital. In reality, a hospital is not the only institution that can fall under the definition of a health system, but it is the most prevalent. Health system is an umbrella term for any institution or practitioner that promotes, restores, or maintains health. Doctors' offices, home healthcare institutions, rehabilitation institutions, and other similar places can also be called health systems. The term *hospital* is still widely used to describe a facility that has patients and delivers care and treatment for the community. Hospitals vary in terms of size, type of care provided, and whether it is a private or government managed institution.

Working or studying in a hospital can be an intimidating experience at first. There are numerous departments, acronyms, and potentially hundreds of employees to interact with. Even learning one's way around the sometimes labyrinth-like hallways can be a daunting prospect. By learning a little about the different areas and departments that exist besides pharmacy, a new technician will have a stronger foundation when entering the hospital workforce. This part of the chapter will help to build an understanding of the hospital as a whole, and also some concepts that affect departments within the facility.

Geographic Layout

The architectural design of a hospital can vary greatly depending on aesthetics, size, location, and the like. Some hospitals may have only two floors (**Figure 1-4**), whereas other facilities may have eight (**Figure 1-5**). Regardless of size, there are some universal principles that apply to all hospitals in terms of layout and function.

Care Units

These areas of the hospital are where patients who are admitted to the facility are cared for. The naming conventions for different units, or areas, can vary, but usually utilize the floor the unit is on, as well as the compass direction of the area's location in the building or ward designation. For example, 2 North and 3 South could mean the units were on the second or third floor and in the north or south side of the building, respectively. Or a designation could be something like 4 Tower, because it is on the fourth floor of the tower part of the building. Letters may also be used for various wings of a facility, such as G1, H5, and so on.

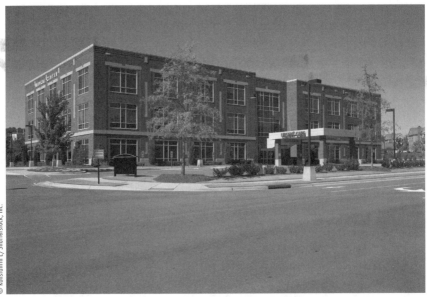

© Konstantin L/Shutterstock, Inc.

FIGURE 1-4 A small hospital.

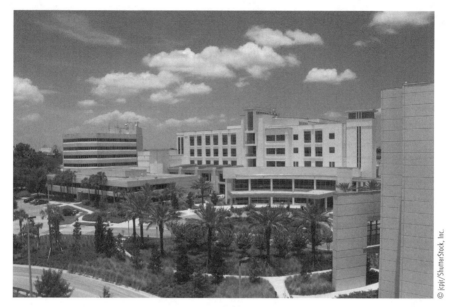

© icpit/ShutterStock, Inc.

FIGURE 1-5 A large hospital.

Inpatient care units also have special acronyms or nicknames based on the type of care received in them. These acronyms are fairly universal. See **Table 1-1** for a list of the most common care unit acronyms or nicknames.

Departments

A hospital is made up of many departments that are responsible for different aspects of care and the running of the hospital as a whole (see **Table 1-2** and **Table 1-3**). A pharmacy technician will interact with almost every department in the course of their work duties, some very frequently. It is important to have a working knowledge of the various departments that make up a hospital besides pharmacy.

Table 1-1 Common Hospital Unit Acronyms and Nicknames

Acronym or Nickname	Translation	Description
CATH LAB	Cardiac Catheterization Laboratory	Cardiac diagnostic and catheterization procedures
CCU	Coronary or Cardiac Care Unit	Care unit specifically for patients with cardiac conditions
ED or ER	Emergency Department or Room	Initial treatment of illnesses or trauma from injury
ENDO	Endoscopy Unit	Endoscopic procedures
L & D	Labor and Delivery	Childbirth and care of newborns
MICU	Medical Intensive Care Unit	Care unit specifically for patients with life-threatening medical conditions
NICU	Neonatal Intensive Care Unit	Care unit specifically for newborn or premature infants who require medical treatment
OR	Operating Room	Surgical procedures
PACU	Postanesthesia Care Unit or Recovery Room	Care unit specifically for patients immediately after surgery
PEDS	Pediatrics	Care unit specifically for children
SICU	Surgical Intensive Care Unit	Care unit specifically for patients after major surgical procedures
TCU	Transitional Care Unit	Rehabilitation unit for patients recovering from injury or illness
X-RAY	Radiology	Diagnostic procedures such as x-ray, MRI, and CT imaging

TIPS AND TRICKS
Location, Location, Location

There is no standard, default layout for hospitals in terms of floor plan. If you were to visit every hospital in a given city, no two would be exactly alike. Even with signs and maps to help navigate, getting lost is still a very real possibility for a new technician. Regardless of layout, there are some common elements that can help when looking for different departments. Certain areas are always situated next to each other, so if you can find one, you are not far from the other. Table 1-2 provides a few landmarks to help speed your exploration of a new hospital.

Table 1-2 Common Departments and Their Locations Within the Hospital

Department or Unit	Geographically Close To
Emergency Room	Radiology, Admissions
Operating Room	PACU, SICU
Labor and Delivery	PEDS, NICU

Table 1-3 Hospital Departments and Their Functions

Department	Function
Administration	Hospital management
Billing	Secures payment for services rendered
Central Supply or Warehouse	Dispenses all consumable products used by patients that are *not* medications
Dietary	Monitors and provides for the dietary needs of patients
Engineering	Maintenance of facilities and equipment, repair needs
Environmental Services (EVS)	Custodial services
Nursing	Direct patient care

SUMMARY

In the last six decades, there has been tremendous growth in the scope of pharmacy technician practice. Technicians have moved beyond the minor tasks of filing, bookkeeping, and other inventory and clerical functions to take over almost every aspect of medication preparation and dispensing.

Almost every duty that does not require the professional judgment of a pharmacist has become the domain of the pharmacy tech. As technology improves and the duties of the pharmacist expand beyond those of a dispenser of medication, so, too, will the roles and responsibilities of a technician expand.

A health system can be a large setting to work in, with many departments and units that are all devoted to patient care. By understanding the designations of different areas, it is easier to navigate the facility with more confidence and efficiency.

REVIEW QUESTIONS

1. What factors led to the creation of the pharmacy technician role?
2. What are some common responsibilities of current pharmacy technicians in a health system setting?
3. What are some of the potential future duties of pharmacy technicians?
4. List five care units or departments in a health system setting and their role in patient care.
5. Where can you find more information about the expanding scope of pharmacy technician practice?

REFERENCES

American Society of Health-System Pharmacists. (2003). White paper on pharmacy technicians 2002: Needed changes can no longer wait. *American Journal of Health-System Pharmacists, 60*, 37–51. Retrieved from http://www.ashp.org/DocLibrary/BestPractices/HREndWPTechs.aspx

C.R.E.S.T. Initiative. (2013). Certification program changes. Retrieved from http://www.ptcb.org/about-ptcb/crest-initiative

Worthen, D. B. (2004). *Pharmacy in World War II*. Binghamton, NY: Haworth Press.

PART 2

Professionalism in the Health System Pharmacy

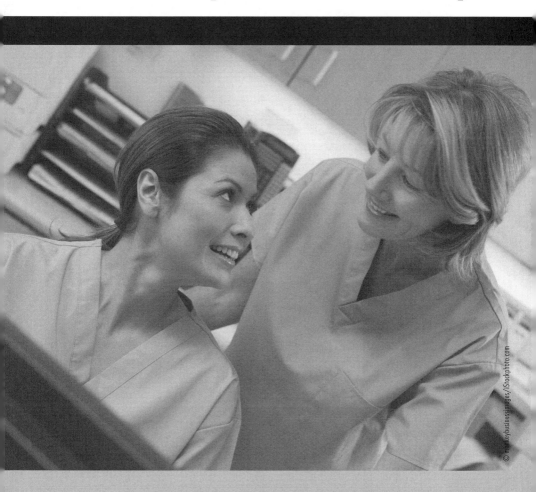

CHAPTER 2

Appearance and Attitude

LEARNING OBJECTIVES

Upon completion of this chapter, you will be able to

1. Identify proper work attire for a hospital pharmacy setting
2. List proper grooming standards
3. Define attitude and mindset
4. Describe proper attitude and mindset in pharmacy technician practice

---

KEY TERMS

Appearance	Grooming
Attitude	Humbleness
Business casual	Mindset
Dress code	Perception
Entitlement	Scrubs

INTRODUCTION

The appearance of a pharmacy technician projects an impression of the quality of that employee. The attitude of the employee complements that appearance. Together, these two traits can be a critical factor in the success of a pharmacy technician. This appearance and attitude not only are representative of the employee, but also are a reflection on the department itself, as well as a reflection on the hospital when viewed by patients and visitors to the facility.

APPEARANCE

Appearance can be defined as the outward or visible aspect of a person. The aspects discussed in this chapter deal with clothing and grooming standards. Every hospital has its own specific **dress code**, or rules for appropriate attire. This chapter will describe the most common standards included in these dress codes for the health system setting. These rules may be stricter than those at a given facility, but should represent at least a minimum standard. If so, it is always easier to relax higher standards than to strengthen lower ones.

Clothing

The types of clothing required for hospital employees are predominately gender neutral, requiring the same types of clothing for both male and female employees. Scrubs are the preferred attire in a hospital setting, but business casual is also possible.

Scrubs

Scrubs are lightweight garments that were originally designed as sterile garb for use in an operating room. They were typically one color, such as baby blue or mint green. They are still used in operating rooms, but now are also worn by nurses, nursing assistants, respiratory therapists, pharmacy technicians, and other health system staff members (**Figure 2-1**). Numerous colors, styles, and patterns are available. Retail stores exist that are devoted exclusively to selling scrubs for healthcare professionals. There are some general rules to be observed regarding the use of scrubs in a hospital setting:

- OR (operating room) scrubs are reserved for operating room personnel and are for use in the surgery department only. These are identified by a specific

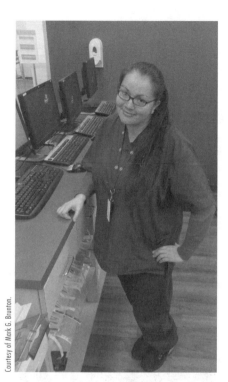

Courtesy of Mark G. Brunton.

FIGURE 2-1 A technician wearing scrubs.

color per facility. A pharmacy technician should have other types of scrubs for use in the hospital, unless their duties take them into the OR on a constant basis.

- Undershirts are recommended, with long-sleeved t-shirts or thermal garments used in cold months and plain t-shirts in warmer months. This is so common that drug manufacturers have been known to produce long-sleeved t-shirts with the name and logo of their product along the sleeves, specifically to be worn under scrub tops.
- Some hospitals have policies restricting or prohibiting the wearing of plain black scrubs in the facility. Even if your facility does not have a policy, it is generally not recommended. Dressing entirely in black can be associated with mourning and funerals, which can be very distressing to patients or visitors to the hospital, where the death of a patient is a possibility.
- Most scrubs are wrinkle free or wrinkle resistant. If there are wrinkles, then they *must be ironed* before use. No matter how nice the material or design of the scrub, wrinkles can ruin the image of professionalism.
- Sagging is not acceptable. Scrub pants should be at hip level *at all times*.

Business Casual

Business casual attire is a style of clothing worn by businesspeople at work that is slightly more casual than traditional formal attire (**Figure 2-2**). Although this is not the most common attire for pharmacy technicians in a hospital setting, business casual clothing is acceptable in lieu of scrubs. This is usually the attire worn by pharmacists and doctors, and it is possible to be mistaken for one if choosing this type of clothing to wear. See **Table 2-1** for a description of business casual attire for men and women.

Footwear

Business casual footwear consists of dress shoes for men and flats or low heels for women. While wearing scrubs, sneakers or tennis shoes are acceptable forms of footwear. This is convenient because the majority of a pharmacy technician's day is spent standing or walking throughout the facility. Therefore, comfort is a major concern. Some notes on footwear:

- Sneakers should be kept clean and in good condition.
- White sneakers are usually standard for healthcare workers who directly interact with patients (e.g., nurses, nursing assistants). It is used to help identify blood spills, but usually is *not* a requirement for pharmacy staff.
- Laces should not be overly long in order to prevent a trip hazard.

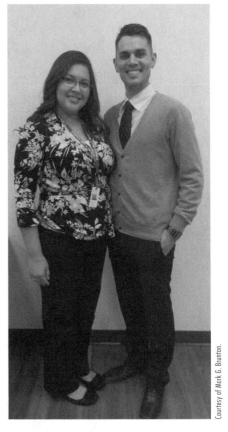

Courtesy of Mark G. Brunton.

FIGURE 2-2 Examples of business casual attire.

Table 2-1 Business Casual Attire

Type of Clothing	Men	Women
Tops	Long-sleeved buttoned shirt	*Conservative blouses or sweaters
Bottoms	Khaki or dark-colored trousers	*Conservative skirts or trousers
Accessories	Tie (optional), belt, and dress shoes or loafers (no sneakers)	*Conservative heeled shoes or flats, minimal jewelry, conservative belts

*Note: Conservative means an appropriate length or cut. For women, clothing should not expose an inappropriate amount of cleavage or leg.

Accessories

In general, accessories such as earrings and other jewelry are not recommended in the hospital setting. If allowed, it is advisable that any necklaces or earrings be conservative in nature. Wedding bands are allowed, as are wristwatches. However, no jewelry of any kind is allowed in an IV room; this is to maintain sterility when preparing IV solutions.

TIPS AND TRICKS
The Value of Shoes

It has been said that a good pair of shoes can increase an average outfit's appearance; conversely, a bad pair of shoes can weaken an otherwise professional appearance. Whether interviewing for a position or working in the department, the effect of a good pair of shoes cannot be ignored. Comfortable shoes help reduce fatigue, which can increase performance and energy. Clean, well-kept shoes demonstrate an attention to detail that conveys professionalism. This does not mean that shoes have to be expensive, however. There are many places to get well-made and good-looking shoes at relatively inexpensive prices. Options include thrift stores, especially for dress shoes, and discount stores for sneakers. Brand-name footwear is not a requirement, as long as the shoes feel good and look presentable.

Grooming

The standard definition of **grooming** is to care for one's appearance. The term is commonly applied to general cleanliness habits. Attire can also fall under this category because it is part of overall appearance. Besides attire, grooming can be broken down into several areas.

Hair

This includes hair on the head and facial hair. Hair on the head must be kept cut according to the dress code of the facility. Unusual hair dye colors (blue, green, etc.) are not acceptable. Extreme hairstyles such as Mohawks are also typically not allowed. Facial hair must be kept trimmed and neat. Goatees, mustaches, and the like should not interfere with any sterility requirements for the facility.

Nails

Facility dress code will have specific requirements for nail length. No dirt should be visible under the nail. Artificial nails are *not* allowed for anyone performing IV compounding operations. The need for a pharmacy technician to make an IV can occur without warning, so it is not recommended in general to have artificial nails if you work in a hospital pharmacy in any capacity.

Facial and Ear Piercings

Most hospitals have a policy on the number of piercings an employee may have in each ear, usually no more than two per lobe for either gender. Small nose piercings may be acceptable in some locations, but other piercings on the face, such as eyebrows or labrets, are strongly discouraged. These types of piercings will have to be either removed before work or covered in some fashion.

Tattoos

Professional standards regarding tattoos are subjective. Dress codes dealing with tattoos will vary in different facilities, with some having no rules applying to them and others saying no visible tattoos are allowed. A safe stance regarding tattoos would be to have them in locations that can be hidden by clothing if necessary. Although tattoos in general have become more acceptable in mainstream culture, it does not mean that all supervisors or locations will allow them. Another perspective to consider is that of the patient. An elderly patient may have a more severe opinion of tattoos, which may impact their interactions with a technician who has them.

Smell

Personal hygiene is always a delicate subject. One of the most difficult conversations to have with an employee or coworker is regarding the presence of body odor. Showering at least once a day is recommended to avoid this potential for awkwardness. The daily use of deodorant should be a standard practice as well. Scents such as perfumes, colognes, or body sprays are to be used minimally, if at all. Coworkers and patients may be sensitive or allergic to these smells. Halitosis, or bad breath, can be mitigated by proper dental hygiene. Breath mints may help mask bad breath, but are not acceptable as an alternative to brushing regularly. It is important to note that an employee *may not be aware* of the fact that they have body odor, because their sense of smell can be desensitized to it.

Caring about one's appearance communicates to coworkers and supervisors a positive self-image and commitment to professionalism. This also communicates to patients of and visitors to the hospital a high level of competency from its employees. This can be viewed from another perspective as well. When buying a car, which car salesman would be more trusted to conduct an honest, fair deal with a customer: The clean-cut person with a wrinkle-free shirt, matching tie, and polished shoes, or the salesperson with body odor, messy hair, and bad breath? Although not 100% accurate, these stereotypes exist and are believed, and a professional hospital technician must be aware of these principles when going about their daily routines.

ATTITUDE

Attitude is a way of thinking or feeling that is usually reflected in a person's behavior. This is a constant aspect of our personality. From the moment a person wakes in the morning until they go to bed, their attitude is visible for everyone to see. This attitude can be positive or negative, and in many instances fluctuates throughout the day. A person's attitude can be influenced by many factors. Some are within the person's personal control, and some are not. Many times the term *attitude* is used negatively when speaking in everyday conversation. "That person has such an attitude!" Or, "Don't give me any attitude." The reason for such a negative perception is that the interactions people remember most clearly are generally the ones that are dramatic or negative.

It is possible to *project* a positive attitude, regardless of how one actually feels. This is a useful trait for a pharmacy technician. The first element in managing attitude is to understand and be consciously aware of the factors that affect it. The following categories are elements that can be controlled actively by any pharmacy technician.

Appearance

When you look good, it is easier to feel good. Rolling out of bed late and throwing on some clothes to get to work on time will look sloppy and make it harder to have a good attitude from the outset.

Time Management

In order to have time to prepare your appearance for work properly, effective time management is a necessity. When someone feels rushed, it immediately affects their mood. When someone has plenty of time to get ready, drive to work, or prepare for an interview, stress levels are lower and result in better performance.

Facial Expressions

Facial expressions are one of the most revealing aspects of a person's attitude at any given moment. They are also generally not thought about by a person at any given moment. One method to use facial expressions effectively is to practice smiling. If you have a negative attitude, it is hard to maintain it if you work at forcing yourself to smile. This has also been referred to in a common phrase: "Fake it till you make it." If a person already has a positive attitude, the conscious effort to smile should not be reduced, and will only serve to reinforce the current emotional state.

Perception

Overall, the state of a person's attitude largely depends on their perceptions. **Perception** is the recognition or appreciation of moral, psychological, or aesthetic qualities. Perceptions can be controlled and managed in part by what a person chooses to value. An example would be the difference between when someone wakes up and thinks, "I wish I didn't have to go to work today," versus, "I am glad I have a job to go to today." It depends on what the person *perceives* to be important.

MISTAKES TO LEARN FROM
When Facial Expressions Go Bad

Once I was talking with an employee about excessive use of profanity in the workplace. The employee was extremely defensive, and launched into a very well-worn argument that held little weight with me, because I had heard it many, many, many times before. As they started, I thought to myself, "And here we go again." What I was unaware of was that my eyes rolled, mirroring the thought as it was occurring (**Figure 2-3**). Although I was unaware of the physical action, I was very aware of its effect. The employee immediately shut down verbally and stormed out of the office. That situation could have been resolved to everyone's satisfaction much more easily if my facial reactions were more controlled. Poker players work on this concept constantly, resulting in the term *poker face*. This same type of interaction can also play out with coworkers, customers, and superiors. I have not rolled my eyes unconsciously since.

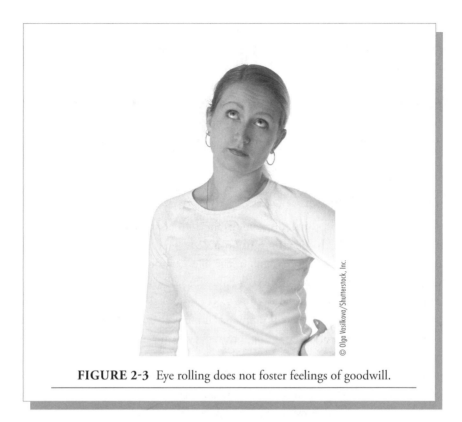

FIGURE 2-3 Eye rolling does not foster feelings of goodwill.

A pharmacy technician's attitude is just as important as other factors in terms of success in the field. Receiving perfect scores in coursework, maintaining perfect attendance, and memorizing drug words do not, in and of themselves, guarantee a job. Conversely, a person who has a fantastic attitude but little retention of pharmacy practice knowledge would also have a questionable degree of success. Only the combination of both will allow pharmacy technicians to truly set themselves above the standard and achieve their career goals.

MINDSET

A person's mindset and attitude are very closely linked. A **mindset** is defined as "A fixed mental attitude or disposition that predetermines a person's responses to and interpretations of situations" (Mindset, 2000). After looking at the prior suggestions for how to manage attitude, a mindset can be considered an overall philosophy or theme that guides an attitude. It can be interpreted as a rulebook for attitude control. As with any new set of rules, it takes practice to adhere to it regularly. The advantage is that these rules or philosophies can be used to work in many different environments successfully. The following sections describe several general mindsets to draw from. These definitions are grouped for organizational purposes based on similarities in concepts. Many of the actions that are initiated from these mindsets tend to overlap and encompass more than one style or type. There is no reason not to explore multiple mindsets, or utilize specific concepts from several.

The Humble Mindset

This is one of the most useful dispositions for both pharmacy technician students and new employees. The definition of **humbleness** is a "modest opinion or esti-mate of one's own importance, rank, or the like" (Humility, n.d.). It is very easy, especially in today's culture, to have a false sense of **entitlement**, or a claim to something. Note the use of the word *false*. The completion of a training program and attainment of licensure are not, in and of themselves, a reason to be awarded anything except a diploma and the opportunity to secure employment. Those mile-stones are merely the key that gets you in the door, where the real work begins.

By developing a humble mindset, the pharmacy technician subscribes to the belief that nothing is guaranteed, and the only way to receive certain outcomes in the field is to earn them through excellent performance. Higher compensation and preferred schedules are earned by hard work and reliability. This has also been referred to as putting in your dues. These behaviors will go far in generating goodwill between the pharmacy technician or student and pharmacy staff.

An application of the humble mindset is the following practice. It is hard not to respect someone who replies to your requests or inquiries with a "sir" or "ma'am." These words can be an easy addition to one's vocabulary. Humility is also necessary when asked to do different tasks. No task in a pharmacy is menial, but the humble mindset can help to ensure that concept is not forgotten. If one is asked to take out the trash, then take out the trash. It may not be medication order interpretation or dispensing, but it is a task that needs to be completed. The phrase or idea, "That's not in my job description," simply does not exist for someone who effectively has a humble mindset.

The Cheerleader Mindset

A cheerleader's goal is to pump up a crowd during a sporting event. For phar-macy technicians, the cheerleader mentality is to always have high energy and a positive attitude, and to try and create that feeling for others in the department. Asking how people are doing, encouraging high performance, and caring about the mood of the staff are activities that fall under this category.

The Hard Work Mindset

Pharmacy technicians who truly embody and believe in the hard work mindset are the star players of the team. They do not complain about the amount of work or variation in schedules that can occur. This mindset is seen in those who will work six double shifts in a row without grumbling, or pick up extra duties without even being asked when someone calls in sick. Many people say, "I am a hard worker," in both interviews and on resumes, but only those who have the hard work mindset will demonstrate this trait in actual practice.

The Switzerland Mindset

When someone refers to himself or herself as "Switzerland," he or she is usually referring to the fact that they are neutral in terms of conflict. This mindset is very useful when encountering differing opinions or methods in the department. The idea of departmental politics can be navigated easier using the Switzerland mentality. A pharmacy technician who utilizes this mindset will not take sides in a conflict, and will be able to work under many different types of pharmacist management styles. For example, a Switzerland technician can listen to gripes and complaints from multiple sides in the department, and each person will feel like the technician is not against them. The Switzerland technician, however, does not offer an opinion on these complaints; he or she only listens. Therefore they are not committing to one "side" or another verbally.

SUMMARY

The measure of hospital pharmacy technicians is not based solely on the amount of drug knowledge they possess, their appearance, or a winning personality. To have the highest chance of success, a pharmacy technician must employ all of these traits in *conjunction*. A successful pharmacy technician must maintain his or her appearance appropriately, practice proper grooming habits, and employ proper mindsets to get along in the department. These traits convey a high degree of professionalism, and are factored into the overall impressions of coworkers, supervisors, and patients in the facility.

REVIEW QUESTIONS

1. Where can you find the dress code for a particular health system?
2. Describe typical appearance standards for a hospital pharmacy technician.
3. What are typical standards for piercings in a hospital setting?
4. List proper grooming standards for a professional technician.
5. Offensive body odor is a sensitive subject. What actions can help prevent this from being an issue?
6. How can a technician display a positive attitude while on the job?
7. Describe perception and how it can be used to affect attitude.
8. Compare and contrast different mindsets in regards to attitude. Which fall most in line with personal existing mindsets? How can this be used to display a professional attitude?

REFERENCES

Humility. (n.d.). In Dictionary.com. Retrieved from http://dictionary.reference.com/browse/humility

Mindset. (2000). In *The American Heritage Dictionary of the English language* (4th ed.). Boston, MA: Houghton Mifflin.

CHAPTER 3

Behaviors and Practices

LEARNING OBJECTIVES

Upon completion of this chapter, you will be able to
1. Define punctuality and how it applies to a hospital pharmacy technician
2. Understand why accountability is important for pharmacy technicians
3. Comprehend the concept of ethics in pharmacy and how it applies to pharmacy technician practice
4. Understand the idea of critical thinking, and how it relates to technician duties

KEY TERMS

Accountability	Ethics
Budget	Punctuality
Critical thinking	

INTRODUCTION

A good attitude and mindset will help increase overall professionalism, an essential trait for a successful pharmacy technician. In order to develop these practices, it is important to discuss the specific elements that go into making a professional hospital pharmacy technician. These concepts and practices are recommended in all types of professions and are especially important in health care. A pharmacy technician's actions and interactions in the field literally have life and death consequences. Proper mindset and attitude will prepare a technician to handle this level of responsibility. This is not meant to scare or intimidate, but only to emphasize the importance of the position.

PUNCTUALITY

Punctuality is the strict observance of an appointed or regular time. When applied to the workplace, this observance deals with not only getting to work on time, but also taking appropriate time during breaks and leaving work at the correct time. A punctual pharmacy technician is ready to start work at the appointed time, does not take breaks for longer than the scheduled time, and does not leave until the end of their scheduled shift. Also note in the definition of punctuality the word *strict*. An employee should strive to achieve and maintain perfect attendance and punctuality *continuously*. The following are some methods to achieve consistent punctuality:

- Get adequate amounts of sleep
- Budget time efficiently
- Expect the unexpected

Sleep

Sleep is critical to personal health and wellness. Lack of proper sleep is a factor related to many health disorders. It also seriously diminishes a person's ability to work safely in a pharmacy setting. One of the major causes of medication errors is a lack of attention to detail, which can be impacted severely by not getting enough rest. Low energy and negative moods are also a result of insufficient sleep. This also affects performance at work.

Although the number of hours of sleep required by an individual may vary, it does not by much. According to studies published by the Centers for Disease Control and Prevention (2011), adults on the average require between 7 and 9 hours of sleep every night in order to function effectively. Individuals tend to underestimate how much sleep they require per night. If it is difficult to wake in the morning, even with three alarm clocks and a significant other trying to physically kick you out of bed, the first step to try would be getting more sleep at night.

Budgeting Time

Commonly, when the term *budget* is used, it is in relation to money. The definition of a **budget** is a limited supply of something. In this case, time is the item in limited supply. As a result, the action of budgeting time is useful in order to make sure there is enough available in order to be punctual and efficient.

The process of budgeting time starts with an honest assessment of how current time is allocated during an individual day. Many times casual assessments are not entirely accurate. How much time is spent getting ready in the morning? Does it really take only 5 minutes to brush teeth and style hair? Or is it more like 10–15 minutes? Keeping a written log for a day or week can help document actual time spent on activities. Once an accurate assessment is made, proper accommodations or adjustments can be made, including finding ways of saving time. This can be done by determining what are nonessential activities, or time wasters. Browsing the Internet may be an enjoyable activity, but if it takes up an hour of the day, that could be adjusted to make time for other, more essential activities.

TIPS AND TRICKS
Time Tetris

Tetris is a classic video game that requires the manipulation of differently shaped blocks to make them fit together without gaps. This essentially is an exercise in how to avoid wasting space. Time spent completing activities can be viewed in the same way, and can be manipulated in much the same fashion. For example, let's say a pharmacy technician has a 15-minute break. She wants to complete three tasks: go to the restroom, order something from the cafeteria, and eat said item. Let's look at the time required for each activity.

1. Bathroom: 5 minutes
2. Cafeteria order: 5 minutes
3. Eating cafeteria purchase: 5 minutes

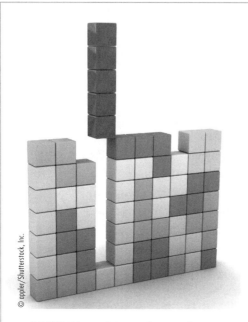

© appler/Shutterstock, Inc.

FIGURE 3-1 Manipulation of activities can yield more time for emergencies.

According to these estimates, these activities can be done exactly within the allotted timeframe for the break. What is not considered in this estimate are factors such as travel time and unforeseen complications. It may take 2 minutes to *get* to the bathroom and cafeteria, and then there could be a line at the cash register. With the current structure of activities, these details would cause tardiness returning from break, and thereby result in not being punctual.

If the technician were to stack the activities differently, much like in the game of Tetris (**Figure 3-1**), she might actually have more time than she realizes. For example, if she were to order the item from the cafeteria and *then* go to the restroom, these activities would overlap. Once returning from the restroom, the order is completed, and there are 10 minutes to eat instead of 5. This gives a larger cushion of time to allow for any additional activities or factors that may occur, and thus maintain good punctuality. This rearrangement of activities can be applied to many areas of practice, both at home and in the workplace. By experimenting with this concept, you will be surprised at how much time can be saved in your day, how consistently you can be on time, and how many more activities you can accomplish in the same amount of time.

Expect the Unexpected

There are always events and factors that are not predictable and can affect a person's ability to be punctual. Although these events cannot be anticipated, their effects can be minimized. Weather, traffic, and emergencies are all examples of things that can suddenly throw off even the most well-planned schedule.

Even though meteorologists seek to accurately predict the weather and give 5-day forecasts to that effect, they are still making *estimates* as to what the weather will be on any given day. The most accurate assessment will occur on the current day. In that case, it is wise to check the weather forecast in the morning before going to work to see if it will affect the morning traffic.

Traffic is in some ways even more unpredictable than the weather, and will directly affect punctuality. How many times have you had to say to an instructor or supervisor that you were late to work because of bad traffic or an accident on the highway? There are many websites that will give an overview of the traffic on your route to work, and even provide alternate routes and estimated driving times. There are also smartphone applications that can give constantly updated assessments of traffic conditions. Utilizing these resources can help you avoid having to explain to an employer why you were 10 minutes late, and therefore not punctual.

Emergencies are the most difficult situations to deal with, and the most varied. A babysitter may be late (**Figure 3-2**), the dog may have scattered trash in the kitchen overnight (**Figure 3-3**), or the interior light was left on in the car, requiring a jump start (**Figure 3-4**). A cushion of extra time budgeted for potential emergencies may help in many instances. Also, for certain events, a backup plan can be created to deal with the emergency. If the car breaks down, an effective backup strategy would be to have two or three people available to call for a ride if necessary, or knowledge of the public transit system as another means to get to work. Although many of these emergencies will unavoidably make one late to work, by using the other tactics listed, this would hopefully be a rare occurrence, or make one not as late as they could have been. It is then more forgivable by an employer, and there is less damage to the overall professional image.

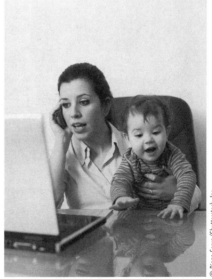

© Diego Cervo/Shutterstock, Inc.

FIGURE 3-2 Childcare can pose unexpected delays and affect punctuality.

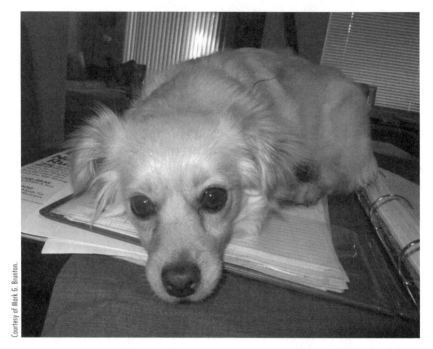

Courtesy of Mark G. Brunton.

FIGURE 3-3 Animal companions can pose challenges to deadlines.

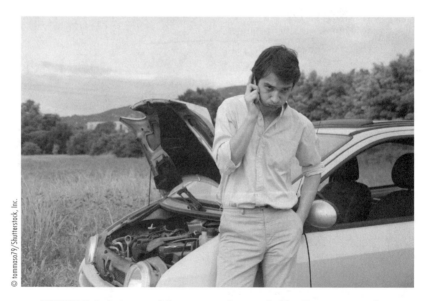

© tommaso79/Shutterstock, Inc.

FIGURE 3-4 Automobiles are not always reliable. Contingency plans should be available when cars break down.

MISTAKES TO LEARN FROM
Punctuality Perception

One of the most common reasons why a student is terminated from an extern site, or not offered a position for employment once an externship is completed, is poor punctuality. This conveys to the employer a lack of reliability or interest in the position. Phrases like, "It seemed like they just didn't care enough to be here on time," are common from supervisors. **Figure 3-5** illustrates the importance employers and supervisors place on punctuality.

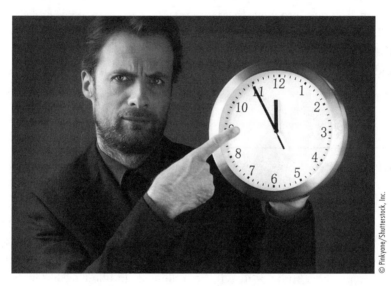

© Pinkyone/Shutterstock, Inc.

FIGURE 3-5 Employers are not always forgiving when it comes to punctuality.

ACCOUNTABILITY

The definition of **accountability** is to have an obligation or willingness to accept responsibility for one's actions. This behavior is one of the most desired in a professional pharmacy technician. Someone who has excuses for everything or constantly blames others for their mistakes does not exhibit accountability. Mistakes will happen in a hospital pharmacy. Mistakes will be made by a pharmacy technician. For example, there will be a time when the alarm clock did not wake someone up and they were late, or there will be a time when a stressful situation causes one to lose their composure. The way we choose to explain our actions demonstrates accountability. More respect is given to a pharmacy technician who admits when they make a mistake and demonstrates accountability for it than one who blames it on something (or someone) else.

Note that in the definition of accountability, the terms *obligation* and *willingness* are used. In terms of patient safety, pharmacy technicians are obligated to hold themselves and others to the highest standards of accountability. There are many instances, however, where it is possible to shift the blame for a mistake or error away from the pharmacy technician who caused it. This is where willingness comes into play. The desire to adhere to these high standards cannot be forced on a pharmacy technician, only encouraged. It is important to remember that it takes *all* pharmacy technicians holding themselves to a higher standard to raise the bar and regard for the profession. It only takes one liar to ruin it.

ETHICS

There are numerous ways in which ethics is of concern for a pharmacy technician. **Ethics** is the definition of what is right or wrong. This concept can be divided into two types: personal and professional ethics. A pharmacy technician can believe things are right or wrong on a personal level and also on a professional one. In many areas, these beliefs overlap. There are some areas where they may differ as well. It is important to examine where these ethics may be put under strain or directly contradicted, and how to deal with these situations.

One of the areas where personal and professional ethics can differ is in regards to religion. For example, there is controversy related to the dispensing of contraceptives. Some pharmacists and pharmacy technicians will refuse to dispense birth control on the basis of their own personal beliefs. In a hospital setting, Jehovah's Witnesses do not believe in receiving blood transfusions. It is then necessary to have alternative treatments available.

In order to reconcile both personal and professional ethical standards, it is important to consider that patient care should be the highest priority. The American Association of Pharmacy Technicians (AAPT) created a code of ethics for pharmacy technicians. These guidelines will help a pharmacy technician in the field make the right decision when ethical dilemmas arise. It is also always good to seek guidance from your supervisor or pharmacy director, if necessary. The following is the technician code of ethics (American Society of Health-System Pharmacists, n.d.):

Preamble

Pharmacy Technicians are healthcare professionals who assist pharmacists in providing the best possible care for patients. The principles of this code, which apply to pharmacy technicians working in any and all settings, are based on the application and support of the moral obligations that guide the pharmacy profession in relationships with patients, healthcare professionals and society.

Principles

1. A pharmacy technician's first consideration is to ensure the health and safety of the patient, and to use knowledge and skills to the best of his/her ability in serving patients.
2. A pharmacy technician supports and promotes honesty and integrity in the profession, which includes a duty to observe the law, maintain the highest moral and ethical conduct at all times and uphold the ethical principles of the profession.
3. A pharmacy technician assists and supports the pharmacists in the safe and efficacious and cost effective distribution of health services and healthcare resources.
4. A pharmacy technician respects and values the abilities of pharmacists, colleagues and other healthcare professionals.
5. A pharmacy technician maintains competency in his/her practice and continually enhances his/her professional knowledge and expertise.
6. A pharmacy technician respects and supports the patient's individuality, dignity, and confidentiality.
7. A pharmacy technician respects the confidentiality of a patient's records and discloses pertinent information only with proper authorization.
8. A pharmacy technician never assists in dispensing, promoting or distribution of medication or medical devices that are not of good quality or do not meet the standards required by law.
9. A pharmacy technician does not engage in any activity that will discredit the profession, and will expose, without fear or favor, illegal or unethical conduct of the profession.
10. A pharmacy technician associates with and engages in the support of organizations, which promote the profession of pharmacy through the utilization and enhancement of pharmacy technicians.

CRITICAL THINKING

Critical thinking is the mental process of actively and skillfully conceptualizing, applying, analyzing, synthesizing, and evaluating information to reach an answer or conclusion. A pharmacy technician in a hospital setting can use critical thinking as a means to solve problems, improve processes, and increase their own value within the department. Critical thinking can also be called "looking at the big picture." By breaking down the definition and applying it to pharmacy practice, we can analyze how to use this process.

Imagining something is the essence of *conceptualizing*. In order to improve a process or solve a problem, a solution must be devised, or imagined, to do so. This solution will come into being by *analyzing* the elements of the problem to be solved. *Applying* the concept and *evaluating* its effectiveness are the next steps. This may lead to changes to the solution, or even the combining of more than one strategy or idea, also called *synthesis*. If this sounds familiar, the scientific method is a famous application of critical thinking, and is an excellent framework to use in developing your skills in this area.

Critical thinking can only be developed with time and practice. Experience is also a factor, because it is hard to analyze all aspects of a problem or process if one is new to a given setting. Once developed and used well, however, a hospital pharmacy technician who practices critical thinking will be the go-to employee for solving problems and fixing processes in the department.

SUCCESSES TO LEARN FROM
Insulin Security Cord

An example of critical thinking used in an actual practice setting was the development of the insulin security cord (ISC) and its implementation in a hospital. The invention and process were created by a pharmacy technician, and were very useful in terms of cost savings and efficiency. To show how critical thinking was used to solve this problem, it will be broken down in the following sections. It is important to understand how the critical thinking process was applied in this instance.

Situation

The hospital in question supplied multidose insulin vials to nursing units to be used on patients by all the nurses on that floor (**Figure 3-6**).

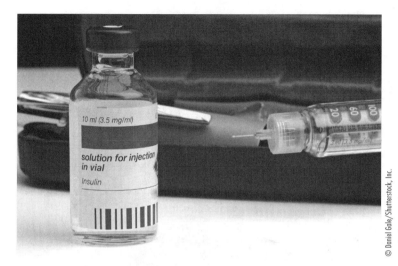

FIGURE 3-6 A standard insulin vial.

These vials were kept in an automated dispensing cabinet, and had to be retrieved by the nurse to draw up the necessary amount. The vial was then supposed to be returned to the cabinet for others to use. The challenge, however, was that nurses would very often take the vial with them to use for other diabetic patients, usually putting it in their pocket. Although convenient for the particular nurse, other nurses who would go to the cabinet would find none for their patient. As a result, the nurse would call the pharmacy to request more insulin. Once a new vial was delivered, the original missing vial was usually returned. This led to frustration in both the pharmacy and nursing department. There were unnecessary phone calls and excess ordering of insulin to meet the perceived demand.

Solution

The pharmacy technician who invented the ISC did so by accident. A combination of circumstances led to the inspiration for its development. While having a cigarette, the technician was complaining to a fellow employee about bringing an insulin vial to three different nursing units, and finding vials already at all three locations. When asking for a lighter, the coworker pulled one out attached to a retractable string, also known as a "lighter leash" (see **Figure 3-7**). The technician jokingly replied,

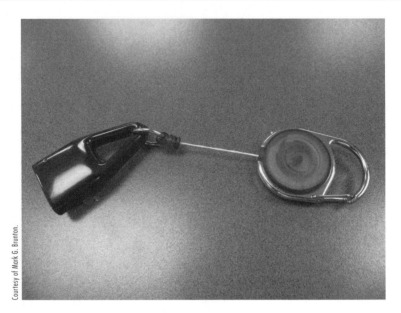

Courtesy of Mark G. Brunton.

FIGURE 3-7 A retractable lighter holder.

"Want to make sure no one steals your lighter, huh?" This is when inspiration struck. The idea was then formed to create a similar device that would attach to an insulin vial, connecting it to a retractable string mounted to the automated dispensing cabinets. This would prevent the vials from being taken by different nurses.

Although this particular solution occurred by accident, with application of the scientific method, the same idea could have been reached intentionally. By using critical thinking, many challenges can be overcome, and the technician responsible will increase their value to the department. Let's apply this situation to the scientific method format to see how this can be done:

1. *Define a question:* Why do the insulin vials constantly disappear from the dispensing cabinets?
2. *Gather information:* Identify the procedure for nurses using the insulin vials.
3. *Form a hypothesis:* If a nurse was unable to take an insulin vial away from the dispensing cabinet, then other nurses would

be able to use the same vial, there would be fewer phone calls to the pharmacy, and less time would be spent replacing missing vials.

4. *Test the hypothesis:* Attach ISCs in several cabinets throughout the hospital. Then record phone calls and replacements from those units versus units that do not have the ISC.

5. *Analyze the data:* Determine whether use of the device proved the hypothesis correct. If so, then implement use of the ISC on every dispensing cabinet. (If data did not prove the hypothesis, then revision and retesting would occur.)

In this instance, the theory worked. The pharmacy department saved money, time, and frustration. The technician responsible was recognized for his efforts and rewarded for his innovation. This process can be applied by any pharmacy technician with the willingness to spend time applying critical thinking and creativity to challenges they may encounter in the field. The very fact that processes are improved in the department makes everyone's job a little bit easier. This itself is cause for great pride and a sense of accomplishment, which can be better than any external recognition.

SUMMARY

When asked to list the traits of their best pharmacy technicians, a hospital director of pharmacy would state the characteristics covered in this chapter. Punctuality, accountability, high ethical standards, and critical thinking skills are traits that all pharmacy technicians should aspire to master. The ones who succeed in displaying these traits are leaders in the industry, and can look forward to a very fulfilling and successful career in the field.

REVIEW QUESTIONS

1. Describe methods to maintain punctuality.
2. What kinds of situations can affect punctuality? Which are controllable?
3. Explain accountability and its importance to a pharmacy technician.

4. What are some areas that a technician has accountability for?

5. Why are ethics so important to pharmacy technician practice?

6. Compare and contrast personal and professional ethics in relation to technician activities.

7. Describe a situation that may challenge your personal or professional ethics in the field.

8. In what ways can critical thinking be useful to a pharmacy technician?

REFERENCES

American Society of Health-System Pharmacists. (n.d.). Pharmacy technician code of ethics. Retrieved from http://www.ashp.org/DocLibrary/Bookstore/P864/Chp1.aspx

Centers for Disease Control and Prevention. (2011, March 17). Insufficient sleep is a public health epidemic. Retrieved from http://www.cdc.gov/features/dsSleep

CHAPTER 4

Interactions and Decorum

LEARNING OBJECTIVES

Upon completion of this chapter, you will be able to
1. Understand the concepts used for proper communication
2. List different healthcare professionals that work in a hospital setting
3. Identify the chain of command and how it affects communication
4. Describe how to communicate in stressful situations
5. Understand "the third eye" and how it relates to decorum

KEY TERMS

Active listening	Receiver
Chain of command	Sender
Communication	Stress
Decorum	Tone
Fight or flight	Trigger word
Nonverbal communication	Verbal communication

INTRODUCTION

In order to work effectively in a hospital setting, it is necessary to identify other healthcare professionals who also work with and in the pharmacy department, and learn how to communicate with them. As a pharmacy technician, you will communicate with every department and staff in the hospital to a greater or lesser degree. Understanding communication theory and its related concepts enables this process to occur naturally and accurately.

COMMUNICATION

There are books, classes, and even university degrees devoted entirely to the science and discipline of communication. Pharmacy technicians should learn the basic concepts and tenets of communication in order to facilitate better interactions within the facility. No career truly exists where you don't have to talk to anyone. There are always other employees that require interaction on some level to complete their respective duties. The function of **communication** is to deliver a message. This message is conveyed through a combination of several different aspects. Some of these methods are sometimes not even consciously used, but they are part of the message nonetheless. In all communication, there is a **sender**, or the person who is conveying information, and the **receiver**, who is interpreting the message. This role switches back and forth in each exchange of the conversation.

Verbal Communication

Verbal communication consists of the words used to communicate a message to a recipient. This is often thought of as the easiest part of communication to control, but how many times do we wish we could take back something that we said to someone? Or how many times have we spoken without thinking? For a pharmacy technician, several different areas of verbal communication should be considered and learned in order to avoid this.

Word Choice

The selection of what words to use when communicating with people in a hospital setting is very important. There are always potential trigger words and phrases that should be avoided, depending on who is the recipient of the communication. A **trigger word** is one that immediately causes a certain emotional reaction in a listener. This reaction can be positive, but in this context is typically defensive. Strong negative emotions can hinder effective communication, and should be avoided if at all possible. Examples of negative trigger words like *always* and *never* can be found in romantic relationships: "You *never* clean the house!" or "Why do you *always* have to have the last word?" A nurse may call a pharmacy and say, "Pharmacy *never* delivers my drugs on time." Be aware of how the words you choose can convey a general observation rather than a specific one. When trying to communicate a challenge, general observations tend to raise less defensive behavior with the listener. For example, saying, "John, *you* never restock the IV room before you leave for the day," may cause a less than favorable response from John. This statement is very specific, and can cause defensiveness. It is possible to phrase it differently: "John, can you help restock the IV room before you finish your shift?" This statement is more general and does not place blame, which can therefore lead to a more favorable reaction. There are many ways to modify word choice to reach a desired outcome. Also, by being aware of which words are triggers, pharmacy technicians can also prevent themselves from reacting to a trigger word. **Table 4-1** contains some examples of negative trigger words and ways to alter word choice to achieve better outcomes.

Table 4-1 Negative Trigger Words and Alternatives

Negative Trigger Word	Example	Better Phrasing Example
But	You may be right, but . . .	You may be right; however, . . .
Never	Nursing never gives their doses on time.	Doses often have not been given on time.
Must	You must answer the phone by the third ring.	It is very important to try and answer the phone by the third ring.
Won't, can't	I won't be coming in to work today.	I am unable to make it in to work today.
Not	That error is not my fault.	I am unsure how that error occurred, but can find out.
Wrong	You're doing this wrong.	This isn't the correct way to do this. I used to do that, too. Let me show you the way they want it done now.
You	*You* forgot to take these meds to the floor.	These meds were not taken to the floor.

Voice Characteristics

The tone, volume, and speed of verbal communication are all characteristics that can be controlled when talking with others. **Tone** of voice deals with the pitch and inflection used when speaking. This can be affected by mood or emotion, which often color the tone. Being aware of which words you choose to emphasize in a sentence is a way of analyzing the tone of your speech. Emphasizing one part of a word or sentence over another can drastically change the meaning of it. For example, the statement, "I don't think that medication was delivered," can be interpreted several ways:

- *I* don't think that medication was delivered: Someone else thinks it was.
- I don't *think* that medication was delivered: It might have been delivered.
- I don't think *that* medication was delivered: Another medication was delivered.

Shouting commonly occurs when angered, excited, or dealing with hearing impairment, but volume control can be a challenge in normal conversation as well. Some people are not aware of the volume of their normal conversational speech, and may unintentionally appear to be shouting at others. Conversely, those with extremely quiet voices are hard to understand. Some people speak

TIPS AND TRICKS
Saving Face

The idea of *saving face* refers to prestige and respect in a group. When there is conflict, saving face allows someone to extricate him or herself from being wrong without losing credibility or respect in the eyes of the group. This concept can be used in verbal communications to achieve better outcomes. By not directly placing blame on or contradicting another employee, that employee may be inclined to react favorably in the future. Basically, do not call someone out for making a mistake or being wrong about something, and they will remember that for future encounters and have better interactions with you. It is a good concept to have in all verbal communications, and can solve many problems before they arise. When pointing out a fault or error, indicating that you have also made the same error softens the critique. This gives the impression of equal footing, and is a good example of helping someone save face.

more rapidly than others, and portions of the message may not be processed by the listener and may need to be repeated. The type of volume that you possess can be examined by asking friends, family, and close colleagues to give an honest assessment of how loud or quiet you actually are when speaking to them.

Nonverbal Communication

When most people think of communication, talking is the primary thing that comes to mind. However, just as important in the process are the nonverbal actions that take place. **Nonverbal communication** deals with the actions of both the sender and receiver that do not involve words. These can be facial expressions, body positioning and movement, eye contact, and other elements. Some tips to improve nonverbal communication that highlight these elements are as follows:

- Be cautious of unconscious facial expressions like eye rolling.
- Good posture demonstrates confidence.
- Avoid habits such as foot tapping, shifting, playing with objects in your hands, and the like.

Listening

Because the roles of sender and receiver are constantly switching between the parties in the conversation, half of the process is listening. It is very easy to have your mind wander while listening to someone, and as a result have poor communication. The need to ask someone to repeat him or herself can be a sign of not being fully focused on the conversation. **Active listening** is a technique to help avoid this problem. In active listening, the listener repeats back the information communicated to them by the sender. This allows for corrections and promotes full attention to the conversation.

HOSPITAL PERSONNEL

Employees in a hospital setting come from a wide range of backgrounds. There is immense diversity in the cultures, ethnicities, and education of the various staff you will encounter. Doctors with many years of education will be communicating with pharmacy technicians with 1–2 years of education. This can sometimes cause anxiety about the proper way to handle these communications. There may be acceptable forms of communication for some personnel that would be completely unacceptable for others. A good tactic to use is to treat everyone with the highest level of professionalism possible. The following is a breakdown of the general profiles of personnel in the hospital setting, and how pharmacy technicians may interact with them:

- *Medical doctors (MDs)*

  Responsibilities: Diagnosing of and prescribing of treatment for patients.

  Pharmacy technician interactions: Doctors communicate with pharmacy in order to determine appropriate medication therapy regimens, including dosing, frequency, and interactions. For these communications, the point of contact in the department is the pharmacist. For technicians, a doctor may call to request access to an automated dispensing cabinet or to answer questions regarding narcotic discrepancies.

- *Nurses (RNs, LPNs, LVNs)*

  Responsibilities: Administering medications, performing certain procedures, administering treatment including medications.

  Pharmacy technician interactions: Nursing is the primary source of communications that the pharmacy handles in the hospital setting. The majority of nursing calls that technicians receive is to locate a medication for a patient. Other interactions can include calling to check compatibility of medications. Another area of communication that is common is in regards to automation technology. Nurses will call to have passwords reset, or to report errors or deficiencies in the stock of a given machine, and to report any mechanical failures that occur.

- *Charge nurses*

  Responsibilities: Oversee Certified Nursing Assistants and nurses on a particular unit or floor.

  Pharmacy technician interactions: Charge nurses will often call pharmacy to inquire about missing medications and delivery times. They may also call with concerns specific to the unit they are supervising.

- *Respiratory therapists (RTs)*

  Responsibilities: Respiratory care therapeutic treatments and diagnostic procedures. This can include administering breathing treatments and breath capacity tests to patients.

  Pharmacy technician interactions: The respiratory department will contact pharmacy to acquire the necessary medications in order to administer therapeutic treatments as requested by the doctor. This request could be for a delivery or a refill of an automated dispensing cabinet, where applicable. If a facility does use automation, these personnel may also call regarding access issues.

- *Certified Nursing Assistants (CNAs) or patient care technicians (PCTs)*

  Responsibilities: Direct care of patients, including assistance with dressing, bathing, and moving. Also responsible for taking vitals of patients (blood pressure, respiration, temperature, etc.).

Pharmacy technician interactions: CNAs may be sent to the pharmacy to pick up medications for nursing.

- *Anesthesiologists*

  Responsibilities: The selection and administration of medications used during surgery to facilitate general anesthesia.

  Pharmacy technician interactions: Anesthesiologists will communicate medication needs to pharmacy, and access issues for automation.

- *Anesthesia technicians, scrub techs, surgery techs*

  Responsibilities: Preparation of rooms and patients for surgery, including assembling equipment, and cleaning and disinfecting surgical sites.

  Pharmacy technician interactions: The operating room will call pharmacy to request necessary medications to conduct surgery. If there is automation in the facility, they may also call regarding concerns of access and function. Direct interaction occurs when restocking the surgery department with said drugs.

- *Pharmacists*

  Responsibilities: Verify pharmacy technician's preparations before distribution to units. They may also consult with doctors and nurses regarding drug therapy. Other activities include monitoring clinical data to help improve drug treatment.

  Pharmacy technician interactions: The pharmacist is the direct supervisor of a technician, so communications revolve around assignment of tasks and verification of work.

CHAIN OF COMMAND

Military organizations are by necessity very strict in regards to obedience and structure. This is in order to maintain cohesion and function in high stress environments and situations found on the battlefield. In terms of interactions, the **chain of command** is a core tenet of this structure. The chain of command is the line of authority and responsibility along which orders are passed. Personnel give orders only to those directly below them in the chain of command and receive orders only from those directly above them.

Interactions between a pharmacy technician and others in the department can be viewed and guided by the chain of command concept (**Figure 4-1**). Technicians who are senior can be considered higher in rank than a new pharmacy technician, with the next step in rank being that of a pharmacist, and then the director of pharmacy, and so forth. This format can be used by a technician when determining whom to speak to regarding concerns or questions; its practice conveys a certain amount of discipline and respect on the part of said technician.

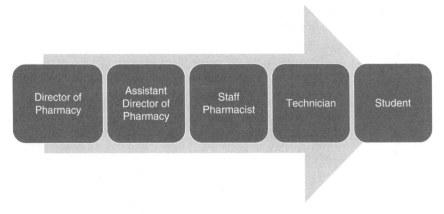

FIGURE 4-1 Chain of command.

Although others in the department or hospital at large may not follow the chain of command, it is better not to follow that example, if possible.

If you are a new employee or student extern and have a question, for example, chain of command can be used. The first person to go to would be the technician training you or one who has been there longer than you. They may know the answer or be able to assist. If they cannot help, or no other technician is available, the pharmacist is the next link on the chain, and then the assistant director or director of pharmacy. Going directly to the director of pharmacy to ask a question about a procedure would be considered a breach of the chain of command. The most likely response to this inquiry would be, "Did you talk to your technician trainer or staff pharmacist about this?"

Unless the place of employment is a military or Veterans Affairs (VA) facility, this concept is not necessarily always practiced or enforced to the letter. There are always exceptions to the practice, such as if you feel you cannot talk to your direct supervisor for fear of retaliation. This is why there are human resources departments to handle those particular types of situations. But for the majority of interactions, the chain of command can be utilized for efficient, organized, and professional communications.

STRESSFUL SITUATIONS

Life and death are daily events in a hospital. Any environment that faces that level of stress can be a challenge to work in at times. This is a challenge that can be better engaged when there is an understanding of the nature of stress. Learning what kinds of stresses can be experienced in the hospital environment is important. Once these have been explored, we can assess methods for dealing with these situations to ensure the best outcome.

The Nature of Stress

Stress has many definitions and covers a wide variety of areas, but for the purposes of this text we can define it as the physical and mental reaction to threatening situations. This is often referred to when talking about the **fight or flight** response, which is one of the body's natural defense mechanisms. When there is a life or death situation, the body increases its heart rate, releases adrenaline into the bloodstream, and suspends digestion, among other functions, in response to the threat. This is a genetic survival mechanism to enable a person to literally fight or flee a situation. This reaction occurs in response to not only legitimate threats, but also *perceived* threats.

For example, if a doctor or nurse is frustrated at not having medications for their patient at the right time, they may raise their voice at you on the phone or in person. This may be their method of handling *their* stress. This can be perceived as a verbal attack, and the fight or flight response can be initiated. You will find that under heavy workloads and staffing shortages, and with patients' lives on the line, many employees in the hospital will experience high stress levels on a regular basis. It is common enough, in fact, that there is often a section of a hospital's policies that addresses it. This policy typically states something to the effect that if tempers are lost and voices are raised, it is to be expected in that type of environment. As long as there is a legitimate effort made to make amends once the crisis has passed, then it is not cause for any disciplinary action. There are not many places of employment that basically say, "It's okay if you yell at someone or get yelled at sometimes, just apologize afterward. This is the nature of the business." This is not a license to lose your cool, merely an understanding that sometimes stress levels can be high in a hospital setting.

With that in mind, one thing to note is that a measure of your professionalism is how well you are able to maintain your calm in the face of stress. If others lose their cool, even on a constant basis, you should strive not to. You will appear more professional than those who constantly vent their stress on others. There are many strategies and tactics for managing stress; here we describe some practices that can assist in maintaining a high degree of professionalism in this very demanding environment. It is impossible to remove the stress factors of hospital work, so these tips are methods to manage the stress you may encounter in yourself or from others.

- *Identify the source of the stress in the situation.* By understanding that stress occurs in the first place, we are more mentally prepared to deal with it. Identification of the source allows for more understanding to take place. If a nurse is having a heated conversation with you over the phone saying she needs a Tylenol STAT, this may *seem* like a rather silly request. It may even make you angry that she is upset with you over something as minor as Tylenol. If we choose instead to identify that perhaps a patient is yelling at the nurse for it, then it is easier to understand why the nurse is agitated. If you feel the need to lash out for some reason, identify first why you feel that way. Understanding leads to better management.

- *Don't take it personally.* An angry doctor really doesn't care or know you personally. A tirade on not having the right medication in the pharmacy for their patient's needs is not a direct attack on your character. Realizing this allows you to not lose your cool as easily. Having a thick skin is a desirable trait. Generally, the angry person will move on like nothing happened the next day, after whatever was causing the stress has passed.

- *Take 10 deep breaths; count backward from 10.* Although these techniques might seem like a cliché, the fact is they can have a centering effect on the person practicing them. Focusing on breathing or counting can help reset the fight or flight response, which can prevent further escalation of the stressful interaction.

- *Reframe your perspective.* Much of our focus in daily interactions is on a moment-to-moment basis. When stressful situations arise, it is helpful to adjust that perspective. One method to use as a guide is the 5-year concept. When determining how to respond to a stressful interaction, you can ask yourself, "Is this moment going to matter or affect me 5 years from now?" The answer is usually no. Asking yourself this question reframes your perspective on the situation, and allows for more control of your stress level.

- *Use the stress.* If there is a stressful situation that demands attention, focus and direct the stress, rather than letting it become a hindrance. Let's say the operating room is calling about needing their supplies right away, there are two doctors on hold for the pharmacist, and two technicians called in sick today. There are generally two reactions to this high-stress type of day. The first would be to succumb to the stress. This is usually demonstrated by complaining about the lack of support, being grouchy, and actually doing less work due to all of the extra work that has been dumped on you. A better method would be to look at this set of circumstances as a way to demonstrate exactly how well you can function under heavy stress. It is essentially "go time." This reaction is demonstrated by using the energy caused by the extra stress to work faster, focus attention on activities effectively, and maintain composure.

Although there are highly stressful situations in a hospital setting, they can be managed so as not to be an impossible aspect of your career. There is a sense of pride in being able to handle stress and stressed out staff with calm, cool aplomb. When people refer to great technicians, their traits almost universally include the ability to operate well under stress.

The Third Eye

In the world of theatre, there is a concept and tool for actors to use called the *third eye*. When an actor is on stage, their third eye is a practiced awareness of various aspects of their image as perceived by the audience. The eye is theoretically above and slightly behind the actor's head. Its job is to watch how the actor is positioned on stage in relationship to the audience, how his or her voice is being projected, whether or not they are conveying the mannerisms of the character, and how close or far they are in relation to other actors. This trains the actor to always be aware in the back of their mind of how they present themselves to others (Hennessy, 2013).

This tool can be applied to pharmacy technicians as well, and is highly pertinent to the concepts discussed in this chapter. **Decorum** is an element of etiquette that describes the appropriate social behavior within a set situation. In a hospital environment, these situations can vary depending on who you are interacting with, and the nature of the interaction. A developed third eye is useful in assessing whether you are maintaining proper decorum when speaking with coworkers, superiors, and those outside the chain of command. What is important to note is that you can maintain decorum, even if the other party is not. While you are communicating with a nurse on the floor, for example, the third eye is constantly checking whether you are making good eye contact, have good posture, and are projecting confidence, and that the tone and volume of your voice are proper for the environment. There are times when we are unaware that something we say can be taken the wrong way by the other party or parties. The third eye helps prevent this.

The development of this awareness is not an instant one. It takes time to instill in your brain the awareness of these extra elements in communication. It is difficult to consciously try and develop this skill in every interaction that occurs on a daily basis. A good method is to try to think about using the third eye for 25% of your daily interactions. That is a more reasonable expectation. If this is done continually, eventually that 25% will grow to 100% naturally, and you will have a new skill to help in not only work conversations, but also numerous other interactions.

SUMMARY

Understanding the basic principles of communication is critical in the hospital setting. By understanding not only how to communicate, but also who you can be expected to communicate with, a pharmacy technician is better prepared to handle any situation that arises in the pharmacy. Whether it is face to face or over the telephone, the same concepts apply. In stressful situations, the ability to manage that stress effectively will be of great use to the technician. Development of a good third eye can ensure that all potential interactions are handled in the best manner possible.

REVIEW QUESTIONS

1. List some elements of both positive and negative verbal communication. How aware are you, in general, of these elements in daily conversations?
2. Why is nonverbal communication an important aspect of technician interactions?
3. Identify three professionals that technicians communicate with in the hospital setting. Where do they fall in the chain of command? How does that affect communication with them?
4. Define decorum and how it applies to professional communications.
5. What are some methods to handle stress? How effective are these methods for you personally?
6. What are some situations in pharmacy that could cause stress? How would you deal with them?
7. Explain the third eye concept and its usefulness to a pharmacy technician.
8. Of the listed personnel a technician interacts with, which would be the most challenging for you? The least? Explain your answer.

REFERENCE

Hennessy, B. (2013, March 21). We need a stronger third eye. Retrieved from http://hennessysview.com/2013/03/21/we-need-a-stronger-third-eye/

PART 3

The Pharmacy Team: Functions and Duties

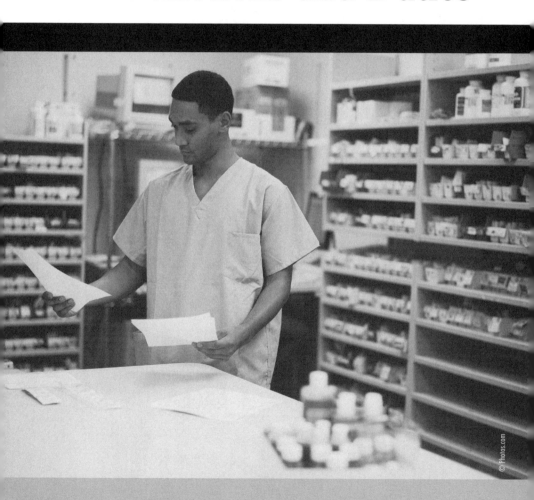

CHAPTER 5

Central Technician

LEARNING OBJECTIVES

Upon completion of this chapter, you will be able to
1. Describe the roles and responsibilities of a central technician position in a hospital setting
2. Define methods to handle various communications with healthcare staff
3. List primary principles of how medications are filled
4. Identify procedures for crash cart refill operations
5. Relate processes involved with anesthesia tray refill operations

KEY TERMS

Central supply   Unit dose
Code cart (crash cart)

INTRODUCTION

The position of central technician in a hospital setting is known by several different titles, including counter tech and main pharmacy tech. The duties and responsibilities vary depending on the size, scope of practice, and level of technology available in each institution. What is universal, however, is that this position is the foundation role for all other pharmacy technician duties in a hospital. A good central technician can support the rest of the team in their responsibilities, but an incompetent tech can increase the difficulty and stress for everyone in the department. This chapter describes the most common activities performed by central technicians, and the methods and techniques to execute them efficiently, correctly, and confidently.

TELEPHONE CALLS

It can be argued that one of the simplest, yet one of the most high-profile, roles of a technician, especially in a central position, is that of answering the telephone. This role can be very intimidating, especially for externs or new hires, but it is one that should be learned as quickly as possible. The efficiency and general level of business in a pharmacy can be assessed by listening to the number of phone calls being taken at any given time. Even more telling is listening to the number of *unanswered* phone calls being received.

A good rule when answering the telephone in a hospital pharmacy is that a phone should never ring more than three times before being answered. A pharmacist in the middle of a complex order does not need to be distracted by the incessant ringing of the main line, and after three rings, may look around to see why the phone has not been answered. Answering the phone quickly, even if only to put the caller on hold, is a measure of your effectiveness as a central technician. A call on hold is a phone that is not ringing. This technique is effective when handling multiple calls at once. Putting calls on hold eliminates the rings. The technician can then begin to handle calls in the order they were received.

When answering the telephone, enunciation is very important in facilitating efficient telephone communications. Tone of voice will also set the mood for the rest of the conversation. There is a quote from the 1980s: "Never let them see you sweat." This adage can be applied to not only telephone interactions, but also all communications in general. Every phone call should be answered in a pleasant, clear, and calm tone, no matter how stressed or busy the technician might be at that moment (**Figure 5-1**).

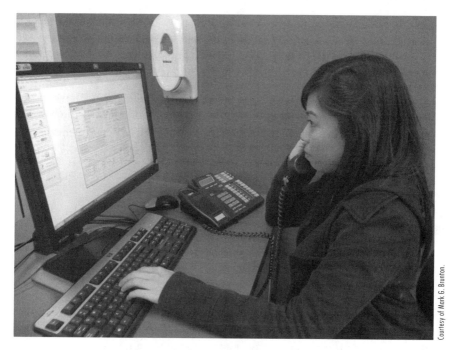

Courtesy of Mark G. Brunton.

FIGURE 5-1 A technician answering the telephone.

The main goals in every telephone interaction are as follows:

1. Announce your name and the name of your department.
2. Identify the caller.
3. Determine the nature of the request.
4. Acquire the necessary information to fulfill the request.
5. Inform the caller of expected time frames and expected outcomes.
6. Follow through or follow up.

Identification

The format of a standard greeting when answering the phone in a hospital pharmacy is: "Pharmacy Department, this is *(your name)* speaking. How may I help you?" Several key elements are offered in this greeting, which can answer some questions for the caller before they are even asked.

Identification of the department is important for a caller who may have dialed the wrong extension, and who was trying to reach the intensive care unit, for instance. The caller can immediately end the call and dial the appropriate extension.

Giving your name is one of the most professional things you can do in your greeting. This simple action shows accountability and responsibility for the call. If callers check back later, they can reference your name to find out the status of a request, instead of saying, "I spoke to someone, but I didn't get the person's name."

Identification of the caller allows the technician to follow up with that person if additional questions arise later. Many times callers will identify themselves, but if not, the technician should ask for their names. The unit or department they are calling from is usually displayed on the telephone's caller ID for easy reference.

Determining the Request

Generally, the nature of the request is stated early in the conversation. At other times, the nature of the request can be vague. The technician should actively listen and ask for clarification if it is difficult to determine what the caller wants.

Acquiring Information

Once the nature of the request has been determined, the technician can ask more specific questions for additional information necessary to complete the request. The amount of information provided will vary from call to call, with the easiest calls requiring nothing more than to say, "Thank you, we will get right on it," and the hardest requiring the technician to take on the role of a detective, asking many questions to figure out the nature of the request.

Time Frames and Outcomes

Once the nature of the request and the required information necessary to process it have been obtained, a good technician will inform the caller of the expected outcome and reasonable timeframe for completion. This courtesy will help to prevent premature follow-up calls checking on the status of the request. This helps to decrease the overall number of calls to the pharmacy.

Follow Through

The nature of the request dictates whether it will be handled quickly or be more time-consuming and involve other technicians and pharmacists. Regardless of the time required or amount of effort necessary to fulfill a request, make sure that it is completed. If the request is handed off to the IV technician, for instance, follow up with that person later to make sure that it was done. If delays occur, follow up with callers to let them know. These actions will promote professional respect for the technician, and improve trust in the dependability and reputation of the pharmacy as a whole.

Types of Telephone Interactions

The following are three of the most common telephone interactions handled by a pharmacy technician:

- Pharmacist calls
- Missing medications
- Technology issues

Pharmacist Calls

Many calls received by the pharmacy require a pharmacist's clinical judgment or authorization to handle. These calls tend to concern contraindications, therapeutic dosing questions, IV compatibility, and the like. The caller could be a nurse, doctor, physician's aide, or other healthcare professional. These calls are usually easy to identify, because the caller will immediately ask for a pharmacist. In that instance, the caller is placed on hold and the pharmacist is notified of the waiting call. If the caller assumes the technician is a pharmacist, they may begin to describe the inquiry. A knowledge of what types of questions are the domain of the pharmacist is essential in order to transfer the caller as quickly as possible, and to prevent the caller from having to describe the inquiry more than once, which is an annoyance that can be avoided. Technicians can prevent this time-waster by stating their position when answering the phone. An example would be "Pharmacy Department, this is Technician *(your name)* speaking. How may I help you?" This practice is common in the retail setting and can be used to great effect in the hospital setting as well.

Missing Medications

Because the main role of the pharmacy in a hospital setting is to provide medications for patients, the most common call is when the needed dose is not available for the nurse to administer. The caller is generally a nurse or nurse manager. Identifying where the missing dose is or what has prevented its arrival to the nursing unit is the method of handling this type of call. The medication may be en route, not available due to shortage, or not yet prepared. Many times, technicians answering this type of call simultaneously pull up the patient profile on the pharmacy database in order to answer the request as quickly as possible. One of the chief complaints from nurses about the pharmacy is the problem of missing medications. A nurse may develop the impression that the pharmacy is generally delinquent in supplying its medications to the patient care areas. In order to combat this perception, follow-up on these types of calls should be a standard practice for the technician.

Technology Issues

Numerous electronic and mechanical devices are in use in hospital settings to facilitate accurate and efficient medication dispensing and administration. When a device malfunctions, be it an electronic order entry system, fax machine, automated dispensing cabinet, or other piece of equipment, if it is related to pharmacy operations, the technician will receive calls when it is not working properly. These calls can also fall under the missing medications category if the technology in question is responsible for medication dispensing. After working in a given facility, a central technician eventually will become familiar with the most common types of technology malfunctions and will know the proper methods of troubleshooting them. Of note is the fact that many people do not like technological improvements or changes and will need clear, easy-to-understand instructions on how to fix minor issues. If the malfunction is something that cannot be solved by the technician, the contact information for the service representative of that particular piece of equipment should be at hand. It is then the responsibility of the technician to call the representative and initiate outside repair service.

Regardless of the nature of the phone call, it is the responsibility of the central technician to screen, prioritize, and resolve issues if possible. It is not, however, the *sole* responsibility of the central technician to do so. Technicians in other roles are always encouraged to assist with telephone answering, if necessary, in order to maximize workflow in the department. It is a good idea to carry a pocket notebook or have one on hand near the phone to write down information as the phone call progresses. Taking notes is much better than asking several times for the same piece of information. This method is similar to the one used by waiters in restaurants (**Figures 5-2** and **5-3**). Only

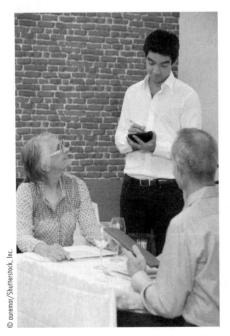

FIGURE 5-2 A waiter taking orders.

© ouremay/Shutterstock, Inc.

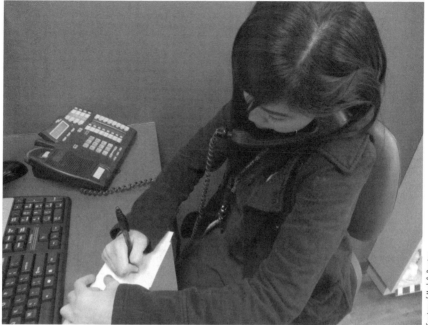

Courtesy of Mark G. Brunton.

FIGURE 5-3 A technician taking orders.

the ones who have been doing the job for many years can take orders without writing them down (and they can still make mistakes), but it is almost a sure bet they started out with an order pad to write on.

FACE-TO-FACE INTERACTIONS

In lieu of a telephone call, a nurse or other healthcare professional may physically come to the pharmacy. The number of face-to-face interactions handled by a central tech depends on where the main pharmacy is located. The author's pharmacy was located in the basement of the hospital. There were fewer face-to-face visits than if the pharmacy were located on the first floor. Processing requests in a face-to-face interaction is similar to the methods used when answering the phone. The main difference is that the person at the window can see you while you are interacting (**Figure 5-4**). It is essential to practice good customer service skills to make sure the person leaves the pharmacy with a positive view regarding the professionalism and service provided.

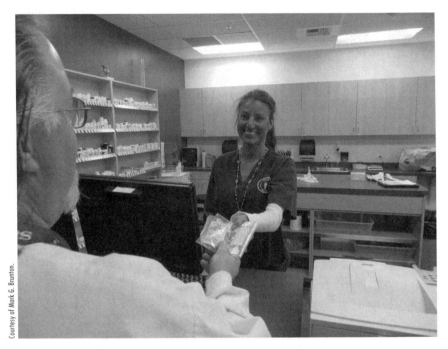

Courtesy of Mark G. Brunton.

FIGURE 5-4 Positive face-to-face interactions in the pharmacy.

MEDICATION FILLING

Another primary responsibility of a central tech is the filling of single orders or doses of medication for delivery to nursing units. Printers located in the main pharmacy generate labels for oral medications, IV solutions, and automation stock notices, if applicable. All medications in hospitals are packaged in unit dose form before being dispensed to a nursing unit. A **unit dose** is a single dose of medication packaged for individual use (**Figure 5-5**).

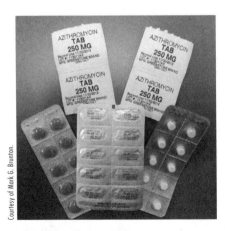

Courtesy of Mark G. Brunton.

FIGURE 5-5 Examples of different unit dose medications.

Labels for patient-specific unit dose medications will usually be packaged in a small zippered plastic bag for delivery. These labels are affixed to the front of the bag and placed in a specified location for the pharmacist to verify.

Different facilities and pharmacists may have different preferences for how to arrange medications for verification. The medication must be either placed inside the baggie before verification or placed on top of the unopened baggie (**Figure 5-6**).

Items in outer packaging, such as ointment tubes or inhalers, have several potential methods of preparation. One practice is to affix the label on the outer packaging, in what is known as flagging. This method is used to avoid obstructing the package label during verification. There is one unfavorable outcome when using this method. The outer packaging is often thrown away after removal of the inhaler or tube of medicine. Identification of the intended recipient of the medication is then impossible. Another packaging method is to remove the medication from its outer packaging, and then affix the label directly to the tube or inhaler. For safe return and reuse, tamper-evident tape is placed over the cap of the medication to verify whether it has been opened on the nursing unit (see **Figure 5-7**). Once it has been verified by the pharmacist, the medication may then be sorted for delivery to nursing units.

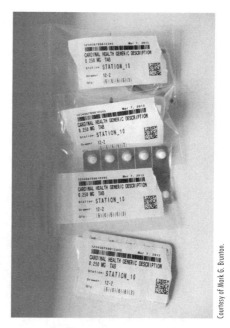

FIGURE 5-6 Doses prepped for delivery to nursing units.

Courtesy of Mark G. Brunton.

CRASH CARTS

When a patient experiences a life-threatening event in the hospital, this is referred to typically as code, code blue, or code 99. A patient in this situation is referred to as coding or crashing. Examples of a code are cardiac arrest and respiratory depression. In order to attempt to resuscitate a patient, a code cart is utilized.

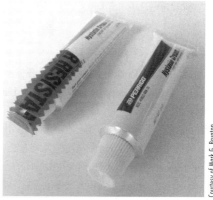

FIGURE 5-7 Ointment tubes with and without tamper tape.

Courtesy of Mark G. Brunton.

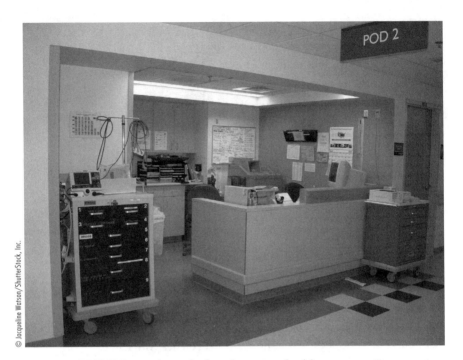

© Jacqueline Watson/ShutterStock, Inc.

FIGURE 5-8 A standard crash cart in a health system setting.

A **code cart** (also sometimes called a **crash cart**) is a portable storage unit of all medications and devices that could potentially be needed during a code event (**Figure 5-8**). A crash cart is stored in every area of the hospital where patients are located. When a code occurs, the crash cart is brought to the patient's bedside for use in resuscitation.

Crash Cart Restocking

The integrity of a fully stocked crash cart is shared between the pharmacy and central supply departments. **Central supply** is the department that provides the hospital with all consumable products used that are not medications, including bandages, syringes, toiletries, and so on. Pharmacy supplies the crash cart with all of the medications required, and central supply replenishes all other equipment and consumables. The technician's responsibility is to replenish medicines that have been used or opened after a code is resolved. The crash cart is typically a rolling tool cart, or built to resemble one. There are several shallow drawers and two or three deep ones at the bottom. In order to efficiently replenish the cart, the medications are stored in removable plastic trays. These trays are covered with a sealed plastic sleeve that is perforated for ease in opening. A *clean* tray is one that has not been opened, and is fully stocked. A *dirty* tray has been opened and may have missing medications. There are several steps to use when restocking a used crash cart:

1. The used crash cart is brought to the pharmacy.
2. Used medication trays and any other pharmacy-specific items are replaced with clean ones and logged for billing purposes.
3. The crash cart log book is filled out.
4. Expiration dates are checked.
5. The pharmacist verifies completion and initials the log book and cart documentation.
6. The crash cart is sealed with a tamper-locking mechanism.
7. Used crash cart trays are restocked for future use.

Crash Cart Tray Restocking

Once the used crash cart has been replenished, any medication trays that are now dirty need to be restocked and sealed. The procedures for restocking a crash cart tray are potentially seen in other operations in the pharmacy, such as kit and anesthesia tray restocking. These procedures can be described generally as charge, restock, check expiration dates, and reseal. Crash cart medications are standardized for every crash cart. A tray from one cart is identical to one from another. A charge sheet is used to document which medications were used during the code. This is for billing purposes and to aid in restocking. The technician fills in the charge sheet of a used crash cart tray by identifying which medications are missing or have been opened. The quantities are recorded on the charge sheet. Replacement medications are then selected and placed in the tray. It is essential that these replacement medications are placed in the correct location and in the correct quantity. Medications are then checked for expiration dates. Note: *All* medications in a crash cart tray should have their expiration date checked by the technician, not just those that are being replaced. A small card can be placed in the tray listing the medication with the earliest expiration date. This facilitates rapid quality control checks at a later date. Once the completed tray has been checked by the pharmacist, it can be resealed in a new plastic covering, and used in future crash cart restocking procedures.

TIPS AND TRICKS
Speedy Checkout

Experienced technicians are able to look at a used tray and quickly identify which medications are missing and need to be refilled by sight. They do not have to use the charge sheet as a reference. This is faster than using the charge form and scanning line by line, checking the names on medications physically in the tray and comparing to what is on the list. Unfortunately, using the charge form is one of the only ways a new tech or extern can learn how to fill a tray correctly. A technique that can help a new tech or student when filling trays is to have a stocked and verified clean tray next to a used one that is being restocked (**Figure 5-9**). This gives the technician a visual reference for comparison, and can greatly speed up learning the restocking process.

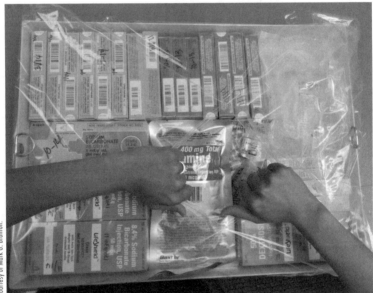

Courtesy of Mark G. Brunton.

FIGURE 5-9 A crash cart tray being opened for use.

ANESTHESIA TRAYS

Hospitals that have surgery departments and operating rooms without automation will utilize anesthesia trays. These trays are similar to crash cart trays in both structure and function. Anesthesia trays have a standard set of medications stored in them that have to be replenished when opened. Anesthesiologists use these trays during surgery to induce general anesthesia, keep patients stabilized, and also reverse anesthetic effects once the procedure is over. The classes of drugs that are stocked in an anesthesia tray include, but are not limited to the following (see also **Figure 5-10**):

- Paralytic agents
- Sedatives
- Stimulants
- Antagonists

The number of anesthesia trays that the central technician has to replenish in a typical shift can vary. The size of the surgery department and how many surgical procedures are performed can affect the number of trays used from one day to

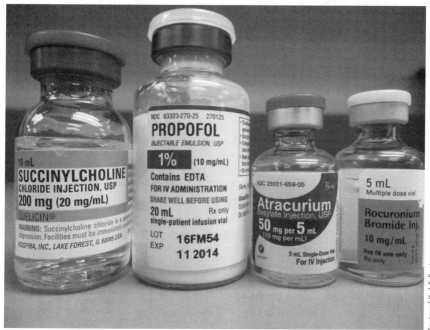

FIGURE 5-10 Common drugs used when filling an anesthesia tray.

the next. The number can be as few as 10 trays to as many as 50 or more. The procedures for refilling are almost identical to those used for crash cart trays, only with different drugs. Because of the repetitive nature of refilling multiple trays, technicians should be aware of the potential for errors caused by inattention or assumption. A sustained effort is required to maintain a high level of attention to detail. What may seem at first to be a minor mistake or moment of forgetfulness could be the difference between life and death for a patient in surgery.

SUMMARY

A central technician has many duties in the hospital pharmacy. The ability to switch quickly between tasks, maintain a calm demeanor, and prioritize effectively is highly prized for this position, especially when it is busy and stressful. From answering the phone or window to filling medication orders and replenishing medication trays, the technician in this role can definitely be considered "central" to smooth and efficient pharmacy operations.

REVIEW QUESTIONS

1. Why is it important to give your name when answering a telephone in the pharmacy?
2. List four of the main goals in telephone interactions. Why are these important?
3. What is the maximum number of rings that should be allowed before a phone is answered by a pharmacy technician?
4. Explain the need for good follow-through practices in both face-to-face and telephone interactions.
5. What kinds of telephone calls should be directed to the pharmacist? Why?
6. What low-tech item can help a technician stay on top of handling phone call interactions?
7. What are some tactics to help maintain positive pharmacy/nursing interactions?
8. What are a technician's responsibilities when dealing with a used crash cart?
9. Why is expiration date checking such an important task for a pharmacy?

CHAPTER 6

IV Room Technician

LEARNING OBJECTIVES

Upon completion of this chapter, you will be able to

1. Understand the concepts relating to IV room operations
2. Describe proper IV room techniques and operations
3. Identify equipment used in the IV room setting
4. Explain various responsibilities in the IV room

KEY TERMS

Ampule

Aseptic technique

Closed system transfer device (CSTD)

Compounded sterile preparations (CSPs)

Compounding

Concentration

Coring

Diluent

Gauge

Lyophilized

Multiple dose vial (MDV)

Pathogen

Reconstitution

Single dose vial (SDV)

Spike

Sterile

Syringe

U.S. Pharmacopeia (USP)

Vial

INTRODUCTION

One of the largest differences between the community and health system settings is the need for intravenous (IV) therapy in the hospital. Currently, a patient would not walk up to their local Walgreens, CVS, or Target pharmacy and pick up an IV for home use. In the hospital setting, however, IVs are used for almost every patient admitted.

There are several characteristics of IV therapy that make it necessary for use in the hospital setting:

- *Rapid onset:* Medication administered via the intravenous route circulates throughout the entire body within minutes, and therefore can be used in very time-critical operations and for life-and-death situations.
- *Infusion dosing:* By setting a flow rate, medication can be given continuously over a sustained period of time.
- *Ease of administration:* Once an IV line is inserted into a patient's vein, medication administration via the IV route does not require any effort from the patient. This is effective in cases where the patient is unconscious, due to coma or anesthesia, or unable to take medication via the gastrointestinal (GI) route.
- *Stability:* Certain medications are too fragile to survive passage through the GI tract before absorption can occur. IV administration bypasses destruction from the digestive system and therefore allows for treatment with that particular medication.

This chapter will explain concepts required to work in an IV room setting. These concepts include an overview of IV terminology and math concepts, equipment and the techniques necessary to use them, and the general duties and workflow of an IV technician.

OVERVIEW

For IV therapy, a patient can receive premixed solutions and fluids that are made by the manufacturer. These are treated like oral medications by pharmacy staff, with little preparation required other than to place a label on the ordered solution and send it to the floor. The other option for IV therapy is when a patient receives an IV solution with medication added to it. This is where IV compounding begins. This is one of the primary roles of the IV technician.

There are many terms and nicknames used in pharmacy practice, otherwise known as lingo or jargon. Many of these terms refer to the same item or concept. This can be confusing at first, but with repetition, you will be able to use these terms interchangeably.

Compounding means mixing. Although technicians may mix many different substances in the field, such as ointments and suspensions, when they are making IV preparations, the term used is *sterile compounding*. When a solution is **sterile,** it is free from germs or microorganisms. Sterility is necessary to ensure patient safety. Because an IV medication is administered directly into the bloodstream, any infection caused by a contaminated solution has life-threatening potential. All of the procedures, rules, and equipment used in the IV room are designed to ensure the creation of a sterile product. An IV pharmacy technician must understand how to make an IV accurately, efficiently, and aseptically to be allowed to compound sterile products.

PRE-PREPARATION CONCEPTS AND PROCEDURES

Understanding the regulations that govern sterile compounding and the math necessary to calculate dosages is required before actual IV preparation can begin. Also required is knowledge of basic IV fluid nomenclature and labeling practices.

USP 797

The **U.S. Pharmacopeia (USP)** is the compendium of standards for medication, food, and dietary supplements for the entire nation. All drugs that are manufactured, distributed, and compounded in the United States must follow the guidelines in the USP. This includes all hospital pharmacies that compound IV solutions.

The USP has different chapters that outline the base standards to be followed regarding different compounds and drug formulations. In 2004, Chapter 797 was released. This chapter dealt specifically with what are termed **compounded sterile preparations (CSPs)**. CSPs are predominately IV preparations, but can also encompass certain other medications, such as topical eye preparations or other substances that need to be made in a sterile environment (American Society of Health-System Pharmacists, 2008).

Chapter 797 is very comprehensive, detailing the proper procedures for a facility to follow if it makes sterile preparations. This includes the design of the IV room itself, employee training and practices, attire, and storage requirements

(Okeke, 2008). When Chapter 797 was first introduced, many hospital pharmacies in the nation were not designed with the standards required. The interpretation of these standards continues to evolve, in order to more clearly identify how to achieve compliance. There are several ways to achieve compliance, depending on what type of equipment and facilities are used. The key to remember is that if a procedure changes, or if new equipment is introduced into the IV room, the reason for said changes is typically to ensure compliance with 797 standards (USP797.org., n.d.).

Anatomy of an IV Bag

In order to work with IV solutions, understanding how to read package labeling is critical. Refer to **Figure 6-1** for the following items (note that different manufacturers may have information in slightly different locations than those shown):

1. *Size of bag:* Lists the amount (in milliliters) of solution in the bag.
2. *ID number:* Used when purchasing solution from the manufacturer.
3. *Name of IV solution:* Describes how to read the name of an IV solution. This is just as important in selection during preparation as using the correct medication to put in the solution.
4. *Solution information (aka the fine print):* This information is not critical for a technician, and can also be found in the package insert for the solution.
5. *Volume measurements:* Much like a graduated cylinder or beaker, these gradations can be used to determine the amount of fluid currently in the bag.
6. *Expiration date:* This is the manufacturer's expiration date for the solution. This expiration date is valid only until the solution has been opened or had a medication added to it.
7. *Lot #:* Denotes the particular batch or group that the IV was made in, and is used primarily for recall and quality assurance purposes.
8. *IV set port:* This is where IV tubing is connected for administration to the patient.
9. *IV additive port:* This is where medications can be added to the solution by the technician.

IV Naming Conventions

One of the most common IV compounding procedures done by pharmacy technicians is injecting an IV medication into an IV solution. The IV solution is the vehicle used to infuse the drug into the body. In order to compound these preparations accurately, you must understand the naming conventions of the

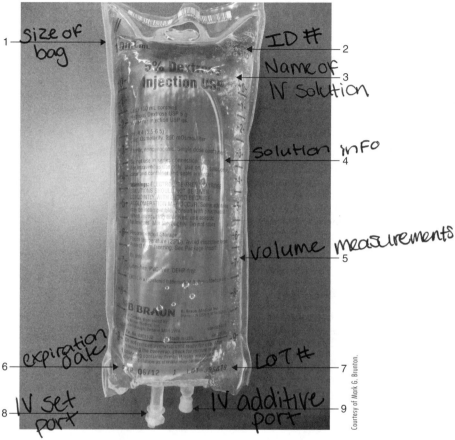

FIGURE 6-1 Anatomy of an IV bag.

fluids used in this process, so that proper selection can occur before preparation. The various IV solutions and additives have many nicknames and abbreviations. See **Table 6-1** for a list of the most commonly used abbreviations for IV solutions and additives. Although direct memorization is one method for learning these nicknames, understanding the rules and general principles of naming IVs will make recall easier. The largest percentages of IV solutions used on a daily basis consist of three main solutions—dextrose, sodium chloride, and potassium chloride—with various derivatives. The key is to be able to associate the verbal or written nickname with what is actually printed on the IV bag to ensure accurate selection and preparation.

Table 6-1 Common Abbreviations and Nicknames for IV Solutions and Additives

IV Solution or Additive	Abbreviation
Amino acid	AA
Calcium	Ca
Calcium chloride	CaCl
Calcium gluconate	CaGluc
Dextrose	D
Gentamicin	Gent
Lactated Ringer's or Ringer's lactated	LR or RL
Magnesium sulfate	$MgSo_4$
Potassium	K or K^+
Potassium chloride	KCL
Potassium phosphate	KPhos
Sodium chloride	NaCl, NS
Sodium phosphate	NaPhos
Sterile water for injection	SWFI
Tobramycin	Tobra
Vancomycin	Vanco

Dextrose

Dextrose is abbreviated as *D*. The percentage of dextrose in the bag is attached to the abbreviation. The most commonly used dextrose solution is 5% dextrose in water, which is abbreviated D5 or D5W. Other percentages can include 10% and 70%. These would be called D10 or D10W, and D70 or D70W, respectively.

Sodium Chloride

Sodium chloride is the primary IV solution used for hydration and fluid maintenance needs without medication additives, and has several nicknames and abbreviations. It can be called normal saline or simply saline, and is commonly abbreviated as *NS*. It can also be listed by its chemical abbreviation, which is NaCl.

Sodium chloride has several percentage strengths, which also affect the nick-names applied to it. Below are the common percentage strengths and nicknames for NS:

- 0.225% sodium chloride: 1/4 or quarter NS
- 0.33% sodium chloride: 1/3 or third NS
- 0.45% sodium chloride: 1/2 or half NS
- 0.9% sodium chloride: NS

When communicating about NS verbally, if no fraction is stated, the percentage is understood to be 0.9%. For example, if another technician asked for "a bag of NS," they are requesting the 0.9% strength; otherwise, they would have specified a different percentage.

Combinations

Dextrose and sodium chloride also can come mixed together from the manufacturer, with the dextrose component being D5W, and the sodium chloride being any of the above-mentioned NS strengths. When reading the label, the naming conventions are the same, just strung together. For example, if a label read 5% dextrose and 0.45% sodium chloride, it would be abbreviated as D5 & 1/2 NS. Because the only two fluids that have percentage strengths and are mixed together from the manufacturer are these two, we can further abbreviate the above example to D5 & 1/2. The NS is understood to be what the 1/2 is referring to. These abbreviations and understandings make communication and label creation vastly more efficient in pharmacy operations. Dextrose can and is mixed with other solutions, such as lactated Ringer's, which would be abbreviated as D5LR.

Potassium Chloride

There is an additional group of IV solutions that consist of NS, D5W, and their various combinations, but also have potassium chloride premixed in them. Potassium chloride is abbreviated as K or KCl, or sometimes K^+. Potassium is a very important electrolyte used often in IV therapy, hence the need for premixed solutions of it. It is, however, potentially deadly if given in the wrong dosage. Because of its possible lethality, any IV bag with potassium premixed in it is very clearly identified by two methods (see **Figure 6-2**).

- *Red box warning:* The color red and/or a bold box around an item in pharmacy labeling indicates important information that should be double

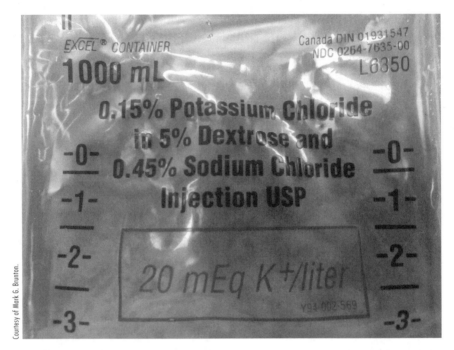

FIGURE 6-2 An IV solution with potassium chloride. Note the bold box for easy identification.

checked before preparation and administration. In this case, the information in the red box is the amount of KCl in the IV solution. The strength of the drug is measured in milliequivalents, abbreviated mEq. The standard premixed strengths of KCl in IV solutions are 10, 20, 30, and 40 mEq per liter.

- The percentage of potassium chloride in the solution is listed as the first line item in the name of the solution. This is placed above the actual solution name itself in order to be easily visible during product selection.

What is interesting about the naming convention of IV solutions with KCl additive is that the KCl is verbally pronounced after the name of the solution itself, even though it is printed first on the bag. Normally when pronouncing or nicknaming an IV bag, the name is read left to right, from top to bottom, just like reading a paragraph. For example:

5% dextrose and 0.9% sodium chloride is pronounced

D5NS

In the case of potassium chloride, however, even though it is listed first on the packaging, it is pronounced last in the naming. It is also delineated by the particular strength of the bag. If a bag is named and has "with 10" at the end, it is known to mean "with 10 mEq of KCl." Although it can be stated in its entirety, the shorter the nickname, the more commonly it is used in the field. For example: 0.15% potassium chloride in 5% dextrose and 0.45% sodium chloride injection USP (20 mEq K$^+$/liter) would be pronounced "D5 and 1/2 NS with 20" as opposed to "KCl in D5W and 1/2 NS."

Size Variations

The last aspect of IV naming conventions involves the size of the bag, measured in milliliters (ml). The most common sizes for IV fluids are 50 ml, 100 ml, 250 ml, 500 ml, and 1,000 ml. In order to indicate a specific size for selection, the number of milliliters is stated after the name. An example would be for a 250 ml bag of 0.9% sodium chloride. When communicating, this would be referred to as NS 250. The 250 is understood to mean milliliters, so it does not have to be verbalized. If no size is communicated, as in "I need a bag of NS," the size is understood to be 1,000 ml, or 1 L.

IV Math

Compounding sterile preparations requires the ability to accurately calculate the amount of drug in milliliters to add to the solution before actually beginning the preparation. This is one of the most challenging aspects of IV production. Once a physical task is learned, such as manipulations in compounding IV solutions, it is harder to make an error, because muscle memory aids in the process. Math, however, has the chance to be calculated incorrectly every time an IV is prepared. Accuracy is essential, because a calculation even one decimal notation incorrect can have life-threatening consequences.

Many "special" calculations are used in the IV room, but are not common in everyday practice. The main calculation needed is the one that will tell you how much of a drug needs to be used to make the IV, based on the strength requested by the doctor and the available concentration of the drug in the pharmacy. There are variations or additional steps in this primary calculation, depending on the particular IV being compounded and how the medication is made by the manu-facturer. In order to understand the concepts of IV math, it is first necessary to discuss the nature of IV medications.

Concentrations

A **concentration** is the amount of drug in a given volume of solution. An example of this would be 4 mg/ml. This literally means that there are 4 milligrams of the drug in 1 milliliter of the solution. The number of milligrams or milliliters used in concentrations varies according to the specific drug. The strength of the drug could be in grams, milligrams, or micrograms, but the volume is always in milliliters. What is important to note is that the concentration does not always indicate the total amount of drug in a vial or ampule, merely how much is in a specific amount of that formulation. This is a constant stumbling block in math problems for students, because it is an extra number given in word problems that may not be relevant to the calculation. See **Figure 6-3** for examples of concentrations on IV drug labeling.

IV Dosing Calculations

IV calculations are required when determining one of two possible types of answers depending on the nature of the order. Most often, a doctor will order a certain amount of medication in a certain IV solution for infusion into a patient. This order will be placed for a particular strength, either in grams, milligrams, or micrograms. In this case, the technician must calculate the amount in *milliliters* needed from the available stock concentration in the pharmacy. The concentration on the medication label is used to determine this amount. Once the amount is calculated, that amount can physically be removed from the medication container and placed into the IV solution. Sometimes the converse is required. A doctor may order an amount of drug in milliliters, and the technician would then need to calculate the amount of drug contained in that amount.

Referring to the earlier concentration example of 4 mg/ml, if a label for an IV requires that 4 mg of that drug is needed in a 1 L bag of NS, no math is necessary. Because the concentration tells us that there are 4 mg in 1 ml, the amount that needs to be withdrawn from the medication vial or ampule is exactly 1 ml. The technician may then proceed with the actual compounding preparation. Often this is not the case. A doctor will often order an amount that is greater or less than the labeled concentration. This is where calculations come into play.

In IV math, as with many other types of calculations, several different methods can be used to calculate the correct answer. No one method is better than another; it is merely what works best or makes the most sense to a given individual. This text seeks to give the most common calculation methods and the rules for how to plug in given numbers in order to reach the necessary answer.

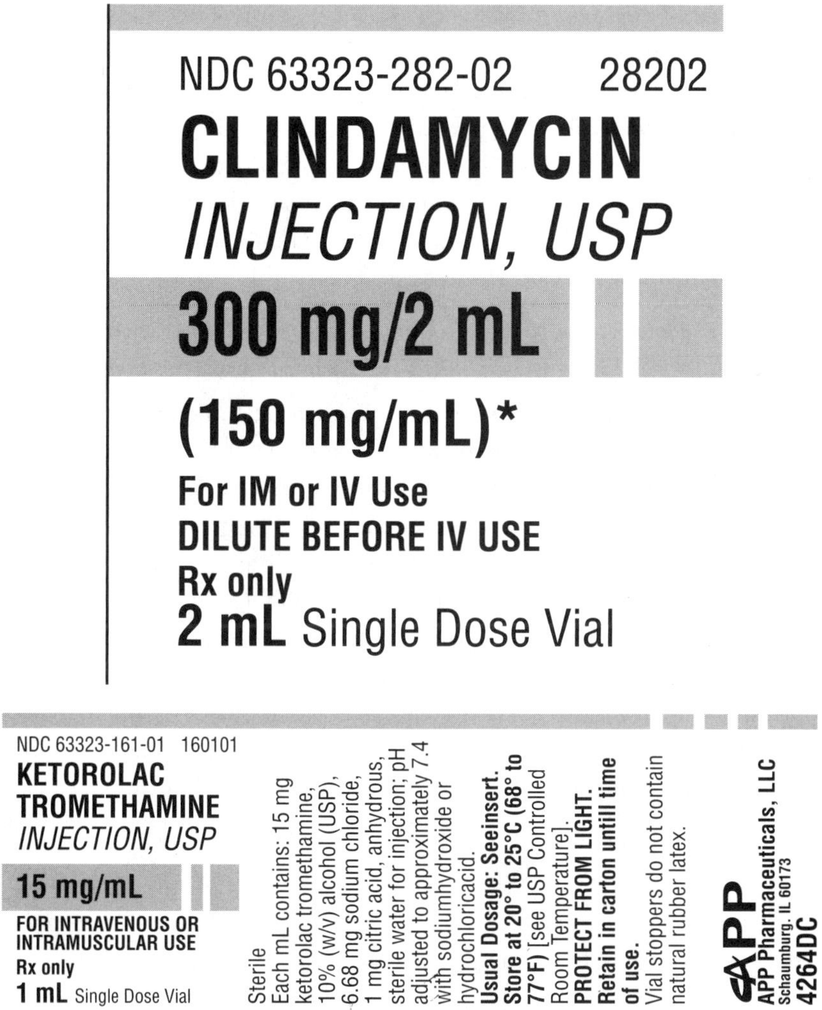

NDC 63323-282-02   28202

CLINDAMYCIN
INJECTION, USP
300 mg/2 mL
(150 mg/mL)*

For IM or IV Use
DILUTE BEFORE IV USE
Rx only
2 mL Single Dose Vial

Courtesy of APP Pharma - Fresenius Kabi USA, LLC.

NDC 63323-161-01   160101

KETOROLAC
TROMETHAMINE
INJECTION, USP

15 mg/mL

FOR INTRAVENOUS OR
INTRAMUSCULAR USE
Rx only
1 mL Single Dose Vial

Sterile
Each mL contains: 15 mg
ketorolac tromethamine,
10% (w/v) alcohol (USP),
6.68 mg sodium chloride,
1 mg citric acid, anhydrous,
sterile water for injection; pH
adjusted to approximately 7.4
with sodiumhydroxide or
hydrochloricacid.
Usual Dosage: Seeinsert.
Store at 20° to 25°C (68° to
77°F) [see USP Controlled
Room Temperature].
PROTECT FROM LIGHT.
Retain in carton untill time
of use.
Vial stoppers do not contain
natural rubber latex.

APP
APP Pharmaceuticals, LLC
Schaumburg, IL 60173
4264DC

FIGURE 6-3 IV medication labels with different concentrations.

The following are some key points to always apply and be aware of when setting up standard IV equations:

- Three numbers are needed to solve an IV equation—the two that make up the given concentration of the stock container, and the one ordered by the doctor, whether it be strength or volume.
- The measurement suffix, such as milligram, gram, or microgram of the concentration, must match what the doctor ordered; if not, conversion must occur.
- Always double-check your answer.

Multiples and Fractions.   This type of calculation is typically the easiest, and once mastered can be done mentally, with no need to write down an equation, and often no need even for a calculator. If an order calls for an amount that is *greater* than the stock concentration but is a multiple of the stock amount, this type of calculation can be done by knowing one's multiplication tables. The factor of the multiple is applied to the amount to be solved, using multiplication. If the amount of the order is *smaller* than the amount listed, a fraction factor applied, and division is the operation used.

Example 1: A doctor orders 16 mg of a drug in 1,000 ml of NS. The concentration available is 4 mg/ml. How many milliliters are required to make this preparation?

The three numbers needed to solve this problem are 16 mg, 4 mg, and 1 ml. The 1,000 ml is part of the *preparation*, but not part of the calculation. Even though it is listed in the problem, it is not needed to determine the amount to withdraw from the medication vial or ampule. It is merely the solution you put the drug into *after* you have determined how much drug you need. The identification of unnecessary information is an essential trait for solving word problems.

Because the ordered amount is larger than what is listed, multiplication will be the operation used. Next we must determine the factor of increase. Looking at the problem, how much larger is 16 mg than 4 mg? These two terms are used because their terms are the same, that of mg. We would not directly compare 1 ml to 16 mg, because the terms are not the same.

$$4 \text{ mg} \times (?) = 16 \text{ mg}$$
$$4 \text{ mg} \times (\mathbf{4}) = 16 \text{ mg}$$

In this case, 4 is the factor. Now that the factor is determined, we can apply it to the volume amount to determine the answer.

$$1 \text{ ml} \times (4) = 4 \text{ ml}$$

Example 2: A label is printed that says to prepare a D5W 500 ml solution with 25 mg of drug in it. The concentration of the stock drug is 5 mg/ml. How many milliliters will you need to make this IV?

Because the ordered amount is larger than what is available, the multiple must be determined:

$$5 \text{ mg} \times (?) = 25 \text{ mg}$$
$$5 \text{ mg} \times (\mathbf{5}) = 25 \text{ mg}$$

The multiple was 5, so that factor is applied to the volume of the concentration:

$$1 \text{ ml} \times (5) = 5 \text{ ml}$$

So it would take 5 ml of the stock solution to make this IV.

Now let's look at when the dose requested is *smaller* than what is listed on the concentration. Note that in this case, division occurs with the factor, not multiplication.

Example 3: An order is scanned down to the pharmacy for 500 mg of vancomycin in 250 ml of D5W. The concentration of the drug is 1 gram/10 ml. How many milliliters are required to make this solution?

Remember that the measurement suffixes must match in order to calculate. So before we can begin, let's convert 1 gram to 1,000 mg. Then:

$$1{,}000 \text{ mg} \div (?) = 500 \text{ mg}$$
$$1{,}000 \text{ mg} \div (2) = 500 \text{ mg}$$

The divisible factor is 2, so therefore we apply it to the volume amount:

$$10 \text{ ml} \div (2) = 5 \text{ ml}$$

It would take 5 ml of the vancomycin drug solution to be mixed into the D5 250 in order to properly compound the order.

Example 4: The pharmacist gives you a vial of heparin 10,000 units/ml, and asks you to mix a bag of D5 50 ml with 2,500 units. How many milliliters would you use?

$$10{,}000 \text{ units} \div (?) = 2{,}500 \text{ units}$$
$$10{,}000 \text{ units} \div (4) = 2{,}500 \text{ units}$$

The divisible factor is 4, so therefore we apply it to the volume amount:

$$1 \text{ ml} \div (4) = 0.25 \text{ ml}$$

It would take 0.25 ml of the heparin drug solution to be mixed into the D5 50 in order to properly compound the order.

These types of calculations are done on a daily basis mentally by everyone in some form or another. For example, imagine you were at the store, and you saw a package of 4 pencils for $1. If you wanted to purchase 16 pencils, you would buy 4 packages, and it would cost $4. Put into IV concentration format, the concentration of the pencils is 4 pencils/$1. When used correctly, this equation can vastly improve your efficiency in the IV room setting. This type of calculation is only effective when it is an easily determined multiple. If the factor is not able to be determined mentally, the calculation discussed in the following section can solve the problem using a calculator.

Desired over Have.   The previous examples are very effective when the multiples are easily determined, because we know the multiplication tables and can apply them mentally. It is harder when the factor of difference is not whole multiples, whether larger or smaller. In those cases, the Desired over Have equation is one method of calculating proper amounts. In this equation, identification of the proper terms to use is essential, as well as which part of the equation they fit in. The Desired over Have calculation is shown here:

$$\frac{D}{H} \times Q \qquad \frac{\text{desired}}{\text{have}} \times \text{quantity}$$

The **D** stands for desired, or the amount that is requested by the doctor or label. **H** stands for have, or the amount of measure that is available as stock. The have number is one-half of the concentration on the stock container. Which half it is (mg or ml, for example) is determined by which unit of measure is requested in the desired portion. **Q** stands for quantity, or the other half of the available stock concentration. When all numbers are plugged in and the equation is solved, the answer will have the same unit of measure suffix as whatever is in the quantity position. The calculation would be performed on the calculator as **D** divided by **H** and then multiplied by **Q**. This calculation is very commonly used in the field. Let's apply the examples from the previous section to this formula.

Example 5: A doctor orders 16 mg of a drug in 1,000 ml of NS. The concentration available is 4 mg/ml. How many milliliters are required to make this preparation? In this problem, D is 16 mg, so:

$$\frac{16 \text{ mg}}{H} \times Q$$

Because the desired amount was in milligrams, the **H** portion would be the milligram half of the stock concentration, or 4 mg:

$$\frac{16 \text{ mg}}{4 \text{ mg}} \times Q$$

The other half of the stock concentration is 1 ml, so that is the **Q** portion:

$$\frac{16 \text{ mg}}{4 \text{ mg}} \times 1 \text{ ml}$$

Because the **Q** portion is labeled in milliliters, the answer will be in milliliters: 16 divided by 4 and then multiplied by 1 equals 4 milliliters.

$$\frac{16 \text{ mg}}{4 \text{ mg}} \times 1 \text{ ml} = \textbf{4 ml}$$

So, using this formula, we have again determined that 4 milliliters of drug would be required to make the IV as requested by the doctor.

Example 6: A label is printed that says to prepare a D5W 500 ml solution with 25 mg of drug in it. The concentration of the stock drug is 5 mg/ml. How many milliliters will you need to make this IV?

$$\frac{25 \text{ mg}}{5 \text{ mg}} \times 1 \text{ ml} = \textbf{5 ml}$$

Example 7: An order is scanned down to the pharmacy for 500 mg of vancomycin in 250 ml of D5W. The concentration of the drug is 1 gram/10 ml. How many milliliters are required to make this solution?

$$\frac{500 \text{ mg}}{1,000 \text{ mg}} \times 10 \text{ ml} = \textbf{5 ml}$$

In order to ensure proper setup of this formula, remember the following rules:

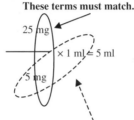

These terms must match.

25 mg

× 1 ml 5 ml

5 mg

These are always the components of the stock concentration.

Ratio Proportion Equations. The following equation is taught very often in the classroom setting. It is closest in its setup to its original algebraic roots. Ratio proportion equations are about "solving for *x*," with *x* being the desired amount. In the formula setup, the given stock concentration is written as a fraction with an equals sign and a fraction on the other side. The desired amount that is given is lined up horizontally to its matching unit of measure on the other side. At that point, solving for *x* occurs either in the old algebraic fashion or using the shortcut of cross-multiplication and division.

Example 8: A label is printed that says to prepare a D5W 500 ml solution with 75 mg of drug in it. The concentration of the stock drug is 6 mg/2 ml. How many milliliters will you need to make this IV?

The given stock concentration is set up as follows:

$$\frac{6 \text{ mg}}{2 \text{ ml}}$$

The desired amount is set as part of a fraction on the opposite side of the equals sign, with horizontal alignment with its matching unit of measure suffix:

$$\frac{6 \text{ mg}}{2 \text{ ml}} \longleftrightarrow \frac{75 \text{ mg}}{x \text{ ml}}$$

Note that the same three terms are used as in the Desired over Have equation, they are just placed differently.

> **Do not mix and match elements of equations, or neither will give the correct answer. Use one or the other.**

The next step is to solve for *x*. By cross-multiplying and dividing, the resulting answer is the answer for *x*. In this example, 75 would be multiplied by 2 and then divided by 6:

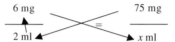

The answer would be 25 ml to compound the order.

Example 9: A doctor orders 50 mg of a drug in 1,000 ml of 1/2 NS. The concentration available is 10 mg/1.5 ml. How many milliliters are required to make this preparation?

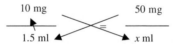

The answer would be 7.5 ml needed to compound the order.

As with other procedures in pharmacy practice, there are multiple methods to calculate IV dosages for compounding. All methods are potentially viable if done correctly and according to the rules for setup and execution of that particular equation. *Always double-check your calculations.* If using a calculator, run the calculation at least twice. Calculators give correct answers only if the information is entered into them correctly. Also, do not ignore the "eyeball" reflex. When looking at the answer to a calculation before actual preparation, if it seems to look off—the number seems either too big or too small—recalculate. It is much better to spend an extra few seconds checking your work than to make a bag that could kill a patient. It is also never a bad idea to have another set of eyes double-check your work if you are unsure about a particular order. People will not think that you are bad at math, but generally will respect your request for a second opinion.

In order to make a 1-liter bag of NS with 16 mg of drug, 4 milliliters need to be withdrawn from the vial or ampule in order to have the correct amount of drug for the preparation. In a classroom setting, math problems are often written out and much time is taken to ensure correct answers. In the field, speed is important as well as accuracy. It would not be realistic to spend 5 minutes on 1 calculation when there are 60 more waiting to be done.

PREPARATION CONCEPTS AND PROCEDURES

In order to physically prepare an IV successfully, a pharmacy technician must understand two core concepts—the identification of equipment used in the IV room, and how to use it in a manner that prevents contamination of the finished product.

Equipment

Numerous types of equipment are used in IV compounding, and newer devices and technology are being developed constantly. Although these new innovations will no doubt make a technician's work easier and more efficient, there are certain pieces of equipment that have been used for many years and are practically universal.

Syringes

The **syringe** is to an IV room technician what a pen is to a writer, or a hammer to a carpenter. Without it, IV compounding could not take place. It is the primary device used to withdraw medication from a vial or ampule and transfer it to an IV solution.

Anatomy of a Syringe.   Knowing the components of a syringe, including what one can or cannot touch when using it, is critical. See **Figure 6-4** for the following terms:

1. *Tip:* This is the location where the needle attaches in order to begin withdrawal or injection operations. The tip can be what is known as either a luer lock or a slip tip mechanism. A luer lock is a threaded shape that allows for the needle to be screwed into it, providing a secure attachment. A slip tip has no thread and relies on friction to hold a needle on, much like slipping a water balloon over a water faucet. It will hold, but can slip off easily when needed. Luer lock technology is used most often for safety considerations and stability.
2. *Barrel:* This cylindrical-shaped body of the syringe holds the fluid being drawn. It has measurements printed on it, much like a graduated cylinder or ruler. These measurements are in milliliters.
3. *Flanges:* These wing or fin-shaped pieces of plastic jut out from the bottom end of the barrel and are used for leverage when withdrawing fluid from or injecting fluid into the syringe.
4. *Plunger:* This part of the syringe is what pushes or pulls the piston in order to withdraw or inject medication.

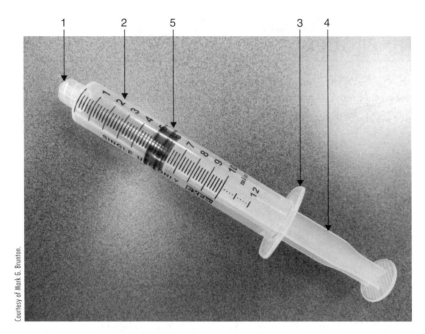

Courtesy of Mark G. Brunton.

FIGURE 6-4 Anatomy of a syringe.

5. *Piston:* This head of the plunger is what seals the interior of the syringe barrel and is used to measure the amount of fluid being used in the barrel. The amount of fluid in the syringe is measured by using the point where the piston makes contact with the inside of the barrel (see **Figure 6-5**).

Syringe Sizes.   Syringes come in several standard sizes, depending on the amount of fluid that needs to be transferred. Syringes come in the following sizes: 1 ml, 3 ml, 5 ml, 10 ml, 20 ml, 30 ml, and 60 ml.

> Note that on some packaging, syringe size can be denoted in cc's or cubic centimeters, which is an older measurement of volume. 1 cc is equivalent to 1 ml.

Once the dosage amount in milliliters has been calculated, selection of the proper size syringe is important. Generally, selection involves choosing the size that is closest to the amount calculated. So, any amount under 1 ml would require a 1 ml syringe, 1 ml to 3 ml would use a 3 ml syringe, and so on. Please refer to **Table 6-2** for an illustration of this concept.

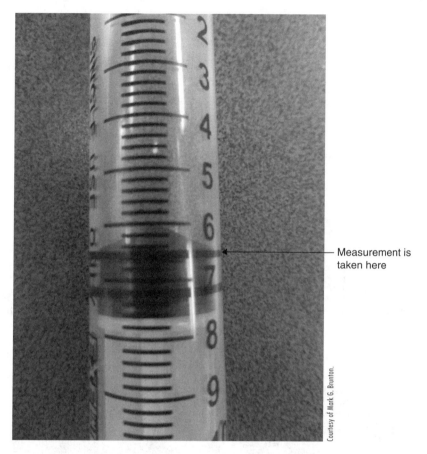

Measurement is taken here

Courtesy of Mark G. Brunton.

FIGURE 6-5 Measurement on the piston.

Table 6-2 Typical Syringe Sizes

Amount to Be Measured	Syringe Size
<1 ml	1 ml
1–3 ml	3 ml
4–5 ml	5 ml
6–10 ml	10 ml
11–20 ml	20 ml
21–30 ml	30 ml
31–60 ml	60 ml

Needles

Needles attach to syringes in order to puncture vials, ampules, and IV bags. Discussed later in the chapter are the ways to manipulate needles in order to minimize the risk for contamination. The good news is that, barring the preparation of chemotherapy solutions, most compounds are not harmful to the technician. This is unlike needle stick injuries in other areas of health care, which are more concerned with blood-borne pathogens from infected individuals being treated.

Anatomy of a Needle.   See **Figure 6-6** for the following components:

1. *Hub:* The portion attached to the tip of the syringe
2. *Shaft:* The body of the needle
3. *Bevel:* The angled tip of the needle

Needle Sizes.   It is important to understand how needle sizes are classified. Two numbers are used when referring to a needle's size: the gauge and the length. The **gauge** is a measurement of how wide the diameter is of the interior portion of the

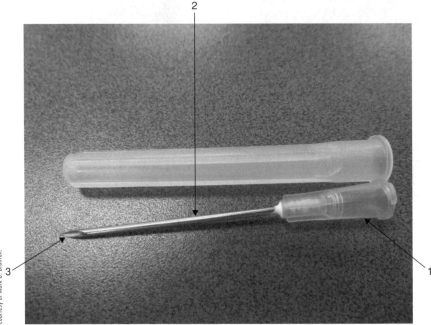

Courtesy of Mark G. Brunton.

FIGURE 6-6 Anatomy of a needle.

needle. The smaller the gauge number, the larger the bore or diameter will be. This is identical to gauge sizes as they are applied for ear-piercing purposes. The length measurement describes how long the needle is from the hub to the bevel. The main size of needle that IV technicians use is 18G × 1 1/2″. An 18-gauge needle with a 1 1/2-inch length is adequate for most IV compounding operations.

For certain preparations, it is easier to use a larger bore needle for both physical comfort and ease of fluid transfer. In those cases, a 16G needle is chosen. These needles are best used when there is a need to transfer large amounts of fluid (>50 ml), or when preparing a viscous solution, such as alprazolam. One thing a technician should be aware of is *when* to use 16G needles. They are not suggested for every operation, even if it seems easier. Typically, fewer 16G needles are kept in stock than 18G needles. It is advisable to use them only when necessary, to ensure that there are 16G needles on hand for the operations that truly require them.

Specialty Needles.   When reconstituting vials of medication, a vented needle can be used. It has air vents built into the hub to equalize pressure when adding diluent. (Reconstitution will be discussed later in this chapter.) Some needles also have tips shaped like mini scalpels or blades, and some have different shapes besides the standard bevel tip. These designs are available to reduce the risk of coring when puncturing vials. One name for these types of needles is Nokor, a play on the phrase "no coring" (see **Figure 6-7**). Filter needles have a particulate filter built into the hub of the needle that blocks particles from being transferred during IV preparation. These are used primarily when compounding with ampules.

Vials and Ampules

IV medication comes from the manufacturer primarily in two types of containers. A **vial** is a glass container with a rubber stopper over the opening. An **ampule** is a glass container with no rubber stopper. Various factors determine whether a medication comes in one or the other, including cost, drug stability, and whether it is a bulk or single use preparation. There are specific items to know about each type of container.

Vials.   This is the most common packaging for IV medications. Vials also may be packaged for single or multiple uses. When a vial has only a single dose, it is labeled as a **single dose vial**, or **SDV**. Similarly, a vial that has more than one dose in it is called a **multiple dose vial**, or **MDV** (see **Figure 6-8**). MDVs have preservatives in the solution so the drug stays viable between uses. It can be punctured several times by a needle, and often is kept in the refrigerator if not

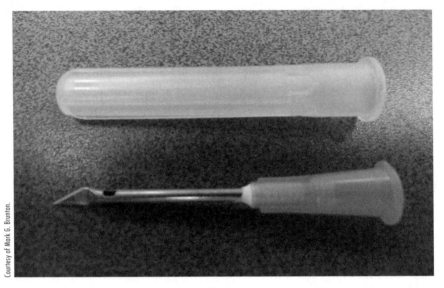

Courtesy of Mark G. Brunton.

FIGURE 6-7 Nokor needle.

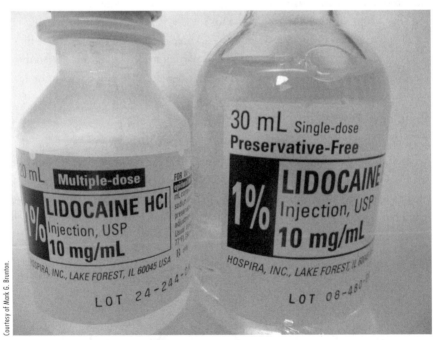

Courtesy of Mark G. Brunton.

FIGURE 6-8 SDV versus MDV labeling.

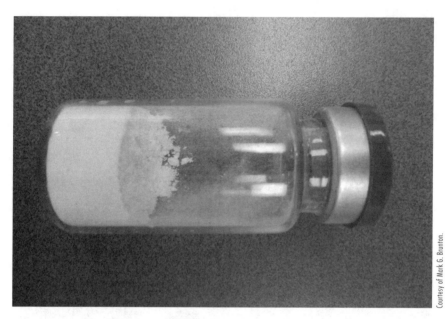

FIGURE 6-9 Reconstitution powder in vial.

used completely in one preparation. Note that when an MDV is kept for use for multiple preparations, usually in the fridge, the date it was first opened and/or the expiration date are written by the technician on the vial. This is so that other technicians who may use the vial know if it is still good.

Vials can come packaged from the manufacturer with solution in them, or as a powder. When a vial contains a powder, it is **lyophilized**, or freeze-dried medication (see **Figure 6-9**). This form extends the expiration date of the medication, as well as its stability. In order to withdraw the amount of drug needed for an IV order, a technician must first reconstitute the medication. **Reconstitution** is the process of adding a diluent to a lyophilized powder to turn it into a solution. A **diluent** is any liquid that is used to dissolve a solid into a solution. This is like adding water to a packet of Kool-Aid. The label on the vial often has the information on how much diluent to use, and what kind. For reconstitution, the standard solutions used for diluent are sterile water for injection (SWFI), 0.9% sodium chloride, or 5% dextrose. If the necessary information is not available on the label, it can be found in the package insert for the medication.

Ampules. Ampules are containers made completely out of glass, with no rubber stopper (see **Figure 6-10**). There is a narrow neck between the tip and body

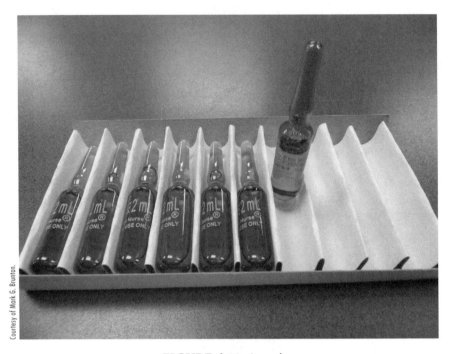

Courtesy of Mark G. Brunton.

FIGURE 6-10 Ampules.

of the container. In order to withdraw medication, the ampule must be opened by breaking it. This process will be described later in the chapter. Unlike vials, ampules cannot be stored for later use in a refrigerator. Once it is opened, the contents must be used immediately, and any medication not used must be discarded.

IVA Seals

Another name for a compounded IV is an intravenous admixture, or IVA. IVA seals are foil stickers that are placed over the port on an IV bag after it has been punctured by a needle (see **Figure 6-11**). This forms a temporary cover or lid to help prevent contamination during transport. These seals can also be used on vials to cover the rubber

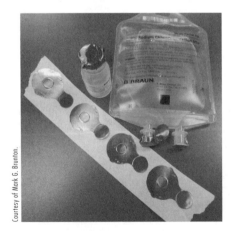

Courtesy of Mark G. Brunton.

FIGURE 6-11 IVA seals.

stopper when it is being stored for later use. These seals are packaged much like auxiliary labels, with a roll of stickers the technician can peel from on an as-needed basis.

Spike Adapters

A **spike** is the term used for a short, very large plastic needle. It is the component of IV tubing that is used to puncture the IV set port for administration to a patient. It is designed to stay in the port once punctured,

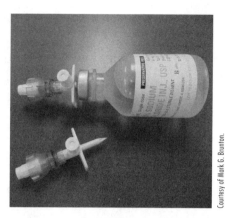

Courtesy of Mark G. Brunton.

FIGURE 6-12 Spike adapters.

and facilitate smooth fluid transfer. A spike adapter is a spike with a luer lock attachment on the other end (see **Figure 6-12**). This device can be used to puncture a vial or bulk IV container and be left in. Any fluid withdrawals from the container after it has been spiked do not require a needle; the syringe is attached directly to the adapter via the luer lock mechanism.

Closed System Transfer Devices

Many IV medications in the hospital setting utilize standardized doses, which means that the same dose is given to a majority of patients for that drug. For example, let's say 10 patients have infections in the emergency room, and the doctor writes an order for vancomycin for all of them. The dose for the vancomycin could be 1 gram every 12 hours for all of them. Because of this standardization, manufacturers package IV medications along those lines. The pharmacy can purchase many 1-gram vials of vancomycin, because that is a common dose. This allows for less waste, because the entire vial is used most of the time. The fluid it is mixed in is also standardized. For standardized IV preparations that are used frequently, closed system transfer devices are a viable option to increase efficiency, save money, and keep up with heavy workloads.

A **closed system transfer device (CSTD)** is a generic term for any device that connects a vial of medication with the fluid it will be mixed in, *without* actually mixing them (**Figures 6-13, 6-14,** and **6-15**). Once an IV has been compounded by a pharmacy technician, the expiration date is shortened significantly, according to USP 797 specifications. This new expiration date could be as short as

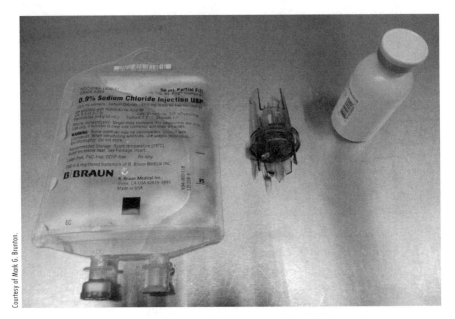

Courtesy of Mark G. Brunton.

FIGURE 6-13 Components of a CSTD.

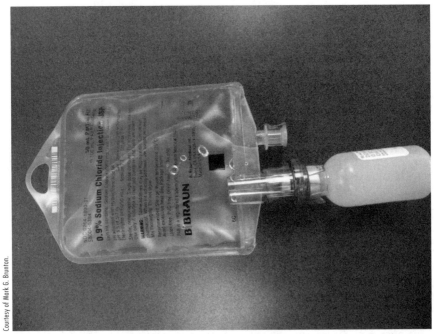

Courtesy of Mark G. Brunton.

FIGURE 6-14 An assembled CSTD.

24 hours or up to 7 days, depending on storage conditions and the nature of the preparation. This means that if an IV is compounded and not used within that time frame, it is discarded. A CSTD is an adapter that has a spike on both ends that attach to the vial and IV bag, respectively. There is a mechanism that prevents the two fluids from coming into contact with each other, but it is able to be activated when the IV is ready to be administered. This enables a longer expiration date, which could be anywhere from a month to the earliest expiration date of the manufacturer for the attached components, which could be a year or more.

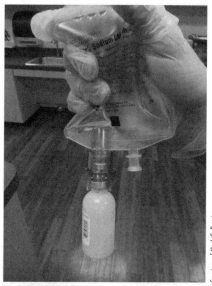

FIGURE 6-15 Activation of a CSTD.

The CSTD is activated by the nurse at the time of medication administration. If it is not used, it may be returned to the pharmacy for credit and reissued to another patient.

There are many brands of CSTD on the market, but many have the word "add" in the name, such as Add-Ease, Addvantage, and Add-a-Vial.

Aseptic Technique

Aseptic technique refers to the procedures that are used when compounding IV preparations in order to prevent contamination of the product. Good technique is demonstrated by the manner in which a technician manipulates their equipment during compounding, and the degree to which they maintain cleanliness while working in a sterile environment.

It is very important to understand the need for practicing good aseptic technique, in terms of the negative impact for patients. For example, if there is particulate matter in a preparation, such as a piece of the rubber stopper from an IV vial, the result could be a pulmonary embolism or stroke, both of which could be fatal. If bacteria are present in a preparation, severe sepsis can occur, which is an infection of numerous body systems. This can lead to organ failure and potentially death.

This section describes the methods used to ensure proper aseptic technique while preparing IV products, in order to avoid these risks. Note that there are

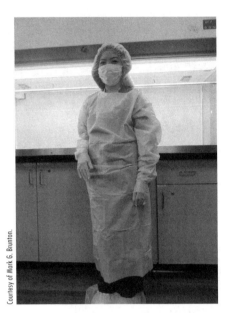

Courtesy of Mark G. Brunton.

FIGURE 6-16 A fully garbed IV technician.

variations of the techniques described; none is any better or worse than another per se, as long as the sterility of the preparation is not compromised. It is then a choice of which variation works best for a given technician.

Garbing

Before a pharmacy technician can begin to compound an IV, they must wash their hands properly, and then put on sterile garb that is free from lint and particulate matter. This garb generally consists of a gown, shoe covers, and a hair covering, but may also include eyewear and a surgical mask (**Figure 6-16**). USP 797 has detailed descriptions of proper attire and garbing procedures. The order of which items should be put on first may vary based on location. USP 797 can be open to interpretation in certain areas, such as garbing. The logic for garbing order is typically based on dirtiest to cleanest items. An example of a common garbing order would be the following:

1. Shoe covers
2. Hair cover
3. Face mask
4. Gown
5. Gloves

Vial Transfers

To withdraw fluid from a vial, it must be punctured with a needle in such a way as to prevent coring. **Coring** is when a piece of the rubber stopper is separated and falls into the solution. If not observed, this particle of rubber can make its way into the final preparation, which could then be infused into the body. To minimize this outcome, the needle must be positioned with the bevel facing up, inserted at a 45-degree angle, brought to a 90-degree position, and then fully inserted into the vial. This technique helps to make sure that the needle is penetrating the rubber stopper in such a way as to avoid coring.

For syringe manipulations, it is recommended to hold one as you would a pencil, at least for needle insertion operations (**Figure 6-17**). The muscles of the hand have already had many years of experience with writing, and therefore very fine motor control can be expected when holding a syringe in the same fashion. This will allow for greater control of the needle during injection procedures.

Ampule Transfers

To gain access to the medication in an ampule, it must be broken open. When doing so, it is advisable to hold the top of the ampule with a piece of gauze to avoid cuts from the glass of the ampule after it is broken. Many technicians in practice do not use this (**Figure 6-18**), because they have a great amount of experience

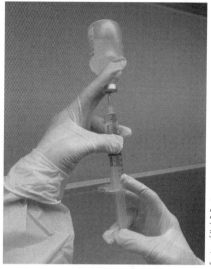

FIGURE 6-17 Syringe manipulation.

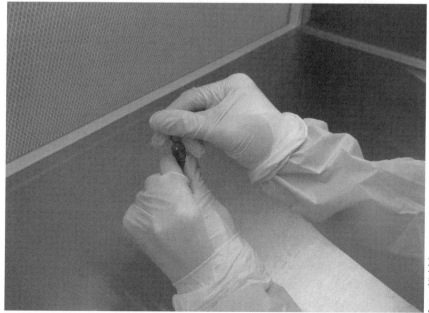

FIGURE 6-18 Breaking an ampule.

with how to cleanly open an ampule. Use gauze until you feel confident in your skill. Withdrawal of the contents can be done with a regular needle. *It is absolutely necessary that the regular needle be switched with a filter needle before injection into the IV solution.* A filter needle can be used for withdrawal, but then must be switched with a regular needle prior to injection. The end goal is to prevent glass particles from getting into the final preparation, and from there into a patient's vein.

Vial Reconstitution

This process is identical to the regular vial transfer operation, except with an extra step prior to withdrawal. A diluent must be injected into the vial for reconstitution before withdrawal. The lyophilized powder must be allowed to dissolve into a liquid solution before withdrawal. The time it takes a drug to reconstitute can be almost instantaneous, or it could take upwards of 15 minutes or more. To help facilitate speedier reconstitution, rolling of the medication vial is suggested. Rolling is taking a vial, placing it between two hands, and rolling it back and forth, similar to trying to start a fire with two sticks. There are some forms of automation available that will roll vials for the technician. *Do not* shake a vial to help it reconstitute faster. Although some medications can be shaken, others are too fragile for that kind of agitation. Unless you know which drugs can be shaken and which cannot, it is advisable to assume that they are all fragile and to not shake any of them.

TIPS AND TRICKS
Reconstitution Made Easy

Some medications are harder to reconstitute than others. These drugs may either take longer to dissolve into the diluents or stick to the bottom of the vial, further slowing the process. One trick is to alter the angle of the needle while injecting the diluents (**Figure 6-19**). Rather than hitting the lyophilized powder head-on, the diluent hits the side of the mass, causing an erosion-like effect to occur. This helps to dislodge the medication from the bottom of the vial, facilitating quicker reconstitution. The steps for this process are as follows:

1. Insert the needle into the vial in the normal manner, starting at a 45-degree angle and moving to a 90-degree angle during insertion.
2. After the needle is inserted, angle it so it is aiming at the bottom corner of the vial.
3. Proceed with injecting the diluent into the vial.

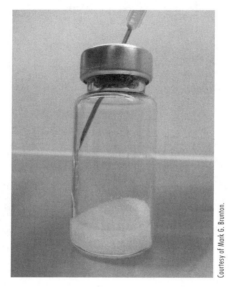

FIGURE 6-19 Reconstitution using the angled needle method.

POSTPREPARATION PROCEDURES

Once a sterile preparation has been compounded, there are several elements still left to complete. The label must be correctly placed on the IV bag, ingredients must be displayed for review, and pharmacist verification must occur before delivery to the nursing unit.

Labeling

The correct placement of a label on an IV bag is very important. With dozens of IV preparations waiting for pharmacist verification, correct labeling can save an enormous amount of time in the checking process. The label must be placed straight and neatly on the bag. Most often the location is directly under the name of the solution as space allows. It should not cover any measurement markings on the side of the bag. It should also be placed with the correct orientation, meaning not upside down. The label should be easily read when the bag is hung on an IV pole for infusion. See **Figures 6-20** and **6-21** for examples of both good and bad IV labeling practices.

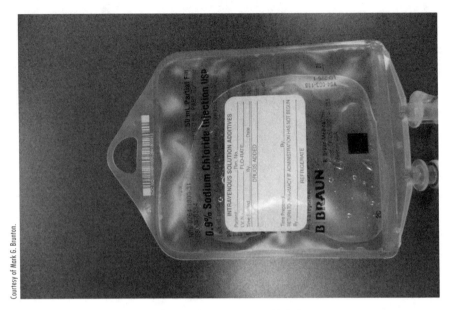

FIGURE 6-20 Proper IV labeling.

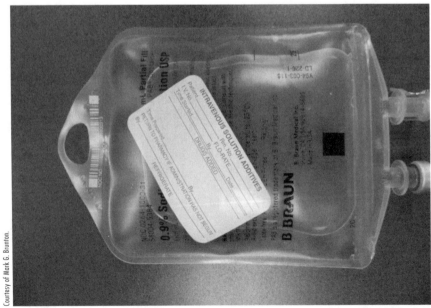

FIGURE 6-21 Poor IV labeling.

Ingredient Placement

When checking an IV preparation, a pharmacist needs to see the original medication vial or ampule that was used in the preparation, in order to verify correct medication selection. One popular method of setting up a preparation for verification is to place the vial or ampule near the top of the bag, and the empty syringe to the right of the bag. The empty syringe is drawn back to the measurement of the amount added. If multiple ingredients are added to a single bag, the placement shifts slightly, with each vial or ampule placed to the right of the IV bag with its corresponding empty syringe placed directly to the right of the medication. This placement is optimal because it falls in line with the natural course of the eye when it reads, which is left to right (**Figure 6-22**).

Pharmacist Verification

Depending on the facility, a completed IV preparation may have both the pharmacist and the technician's initials written on it, or just those of the pharmacist. No preparation should ever leave the pharmacy without the necessary number of

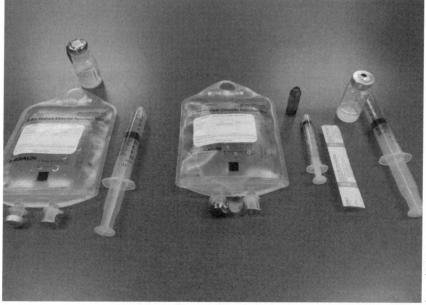

Courtesy of Mark G. Brunton.

FIGURE 6-22 IV laid out for checking, single and multiple ingredients.

initials. Pharmacist preferences vary on the manner in which they like to check IVs, and it is the technician's responsibility to understand them all and be able to use whichever method is preferred on a given day for a given pharmacist. This adaptability is the hallmark of a superior IV room technician.

NONPREPARATION PROCEDURES

Several activities and duties are performed by an IV room technician that are not directly involved in the preparation of IVs. Various quality assurance procedures and logs need to be completed. Calibrations, sterility tests, and restocking must also be performed in order to keep the entire IV room functioning at peak performance. Because these activities are not as time sensitive as IV compounding, they have a tendency to become secondary in terms of importance, or put on the back burner. Ironically these are the areas that accrediting bodies such as The Joint Commission tend to target first during inspections. As a result, these tasks cannot be ignored or put off for very long, and are an area of accountability for technicians.

Temperature Logs

Every refrigerator, freezer, or even warming cabinet in an IV room must be checked at least once daily to ensure that correct temperature ranges are being maintained. If these devices were to break down or fall out of range for a long enough period of time, the medication stored within would go bad and have to be wasted. This theory is identical to having food in your refrigerator that has spoiled because the power was out all day.

In order to document daily temperature verification, a log sheet is attached to the unit, with acceptable ranges listed on it (see **Figure 6-23**). A technician must record the temperature of the unit daily in the log. If a day is missed, a technician cannot go back and fill it in. This is fraud. It is also a liability. If the fridge did fall out of range, any adverse results of potentially contaminated medication during that time would fall on both the technician that did not document checking and the technician who tried to cover up the lapse. It is better to leave a day blank rather than fake it.

The steps to take if a refrigerator or warmer falls out of range are as follows:

1. Adjust temperature settings within the unit. Wait for approximately 1 hour and check temperature again.

2. If step 1 was unsuccessful, notify the appropriate department to fix the cooling or heating element of the device. Typically the engineering department is responsible for refrigerator maintenance.
3. Once repairs are complete, check to ensure the temperature is back in range.

Sterility Testing

To ensure that technicians are maintaining proper sterile technique during IV compounding procedures, sterility tests are conducted. This can be done very often or less depending on the facility, but should be done at least on an annual basis. Documentation of the results is kept in log books to show accrediting agencies if requested. The two main tests used are Agar plate and what are known as broth bag tests.

Agar Plate

Also known as a fingertip test, this test ensures that garbing was completed properly, and that no pathogens are present on the technician's hands. **Pathogens** are disease-causing agents. This test involves completing the garbing procedure and then pressing a gloved fingertip onto a plastic dish containing growth medium (see **Figure 6-24**). The plate is then stored for a specified time frame. The test shows whether bacteria are present on the glove at the time of testing. They will grow in the plate and be visible to the naked eye. If there is bacterial growth, the test is considered failed and additional training may be implemented to correct garbing technique deficiencies.

Broth Bag

A standardized IV sterility test determines whether a technician's aseptic technique is being performed properly during IV compounding procedures. It consists of a 250 ml bag of amber-colored solution, and a 20 ml vial of growth medium. The standard process is to use 1 syringe and 20 needles. The technician would proceed to withdraw 1 ml at a time from the vial and inject it into the bag. The technician would use a new needle each time, but never change the syringe. This simulates the absolute worst conditions possible while preparing a solution. The bag is then incubated in a warming cabinet. If there is no bacterial growth after a specified amount of time, then the technician has demonstrated competent aseptic technique (**Figure 6-25**).

Medication Refrigerator/Freezer Temperature Log

Agency Name

Location: _____

Month/Year: _____

Appropriate Refrigerator Range = 36°F to 46°F
Appropriate Freezer Range = 5°F or LOWER

| Day | REFRIGERATOR | | | | | | | | | FREEZER | | | | | |
| | AM | | | | PM | | | | | AM | | | PM | | |
	Temp (°F)	Min	Max	Initials / Comments	Temp (°F)	Min	Max	Initials / Comments		Temp (°F)	Initials		Temp (°F)	Initials / Comments	Doors closed at end of day
1															
2															
3															
4															
5															
6															
7															
8															
9															
10															
11															
12															

13											
14											
15											
16											
17											
18											
19											
20											
21											
22											
23											
24											
25											
26											
27											
28											
29											
30											
31											

In the event that the refrigerator and/or freezer temperature (including **min/max temperature values for refrigerator**) are not within the accepted range, staff shall **IMMEDIATELY NOTIFY the clinic manager or nursing leader** who will seek consultation to determine if medications and antigens remain viable.

FIGURE 6-23 Refrigerator temperature log.

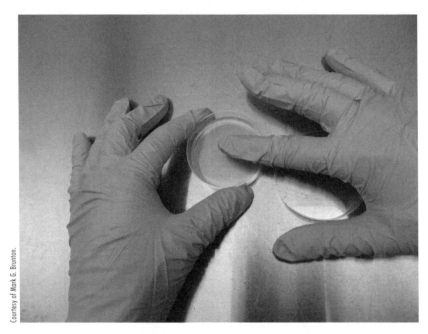

Courtesy of Mark G. Brunton.

FIGURE 6-24 Fingertip sterility test.

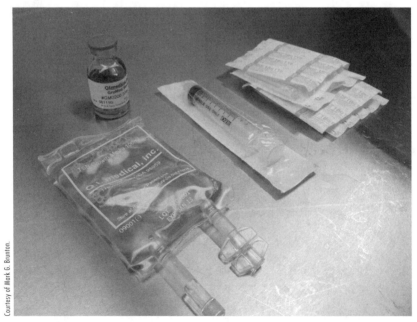

Courtesy of Mark G. Brunton.

FIGURE 6-25 Broth bag sterility test.

Restocking

During the course of the day, an IV technician will invariably run low on supplies. There is usually a storeroom located nearby that has additional cases of syringes, needles, IV solutions, and the like. Refilling all supplies for the next shift is a courtesy that is not to be ignored (**Figure 6-26**). This is a duty of a responsible and considerate technician. Always make sure to leave enough time at the end of shift to gather the necessary supplies that are depleted.

Reconciliation Rounds

During a reconciliation round, the IV technician goes to every nursing unit in the facility and recovers any IV preparations that were not used in the last 24 hours. The purpose for this is twofold. Any IV solutions that are not expired can be reused for the next batch, which saves preparation time. Reconciliation also frees up space on the floor for the next batch, which can be a significant amount of IVs.

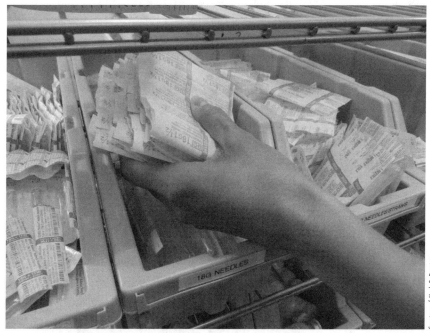

Courtesy of Mark G. Brunton.

FIGURE 6-26 Restocking is a daily function for a pharmacy technician in a health system setting.

Batching

The term *batching* actually can refer to two different concepts in an IV room. Batching as a verb refers to a certain type of compounding done before an order has been placed. It allows an IV technician to stay on top of demand for popular and common IV medications that are used repeatedly and in the same doses. Batching involves compounding many bags of the same drug and dose in anticipation of the order for them. When a label is produced for a batched medication, the technician merely needs to affix it to the preparation that has already been prepared ahead of time, and have it verified by the pharmacist. This is similar to making a batch of cupcakes for your coworkers or family and friends. You don't know who will eat them, but you anticipate that they will all be eaten. The numbers of IVs batched at a given time are determined by historical use of the particular drug.

A logbook is used to document when a batch is made, because there is not an individual patient label yet. The technician fills out the logbook, and a pharmacist verifies that the ingredients and information are accurate. Smaller labels are placed on the finished preparations in lieu of a patient-specific label. These indicate what medication has been added to it, its strength, lot number, and expiration date. These IVs can then be stored for use until they are needed (**Figure 6-27**). Batching can have

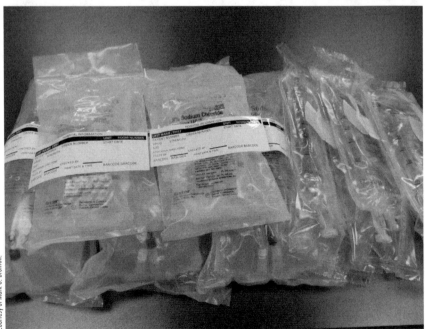

Courtesy of Mark G. Brunton.

FIGURE 6-27 An IV batch awaiting verification and delivery.

an assigned time for completion during the workday, or can be done whenever there is downtime in the IV room. CSTDs are also batched in this fashion and for much the same purpose.

The term *batch* when used as a noun refers to one of the major operations done daily in an IV room. The pharmacy in a hospital setting provides medications for patients on a 24-hour basis. The average length of stay for a patient is 3–5 days, so it is not realistic to dispense enough of an ordered IV to last for a week or month. Orders also change on a daily basis for a given drug, depending on the response of the patient to therapy. At least once daily, a batch of labels is printed from the pharmacy database. These are the labels of all of the IV drugs prescribed for all patients in the hospital. Enough labels are generated to supply the patient for the next 24 hours. For example, if a patient has an order in the computer for a vancomycin 1.2 gram IV q12h, the batch will print two labels for the patient for this drug. The technician can then prepare enough vancomycin to last the patient until the next batch the following day. This is identical in process and concept to a cart fill procedure, only for IV solutions. Any orders or changes to orders that occur after the batch has printed will print out as additional labels, and be filled as time allows. Note that batches are run in 12- or 24-hour increments.

SUMMARY

There are many aspects to be aware of when working in an IV room setting. Many new technicians or students can be intimidated by all of the specialized equipment and procedures required to prepare a proper compounded sterile product. Training for this role is extensive, but with practice, this role can be mastered. The most important notes to remember are to double-check all calculations and physical preparations. It is also wise to acknowledge when you are in doubt about a rule, policy, or technique. Do not be afraid to ask a more experienced technician or pharmacist. One of the best methods to help ensure good IV preparations can be summed up as, "When in doubt, throw it out."

REVIEW QUESTIONS

1. List some of the reasons why IV medications are used in the hospital setting.
2. List three standards that must be practiced per USP 797 guidelines when preparing IVs.

3. Why is it important to understand IV nicknames and other related jargon when working in the IV room setting?

4. Why is correct syringe size selection important in IV compounding procedures?

5. What areas should not be touched when working with a syringe and needle?

6. Describe the proper procedure for withdrawing medication from a vial.

7. Describe the proper procedure for withdrawing medication from an ampule.

8. Describe the proper procedure for reconstitution of a medication.

9. Why do some drugs need to be reconstituted?

10. List some of the benefits of CSTDs.

11. Define aseptic technique and its importance to IV preparations.

12. What is the purpose of sterility testing?

REFERENCES

American Society of Health-System Pharmacists. (2008). The ASHP discussion guide on USP chapter <797> for compounding sterile preparations. Retrieved from http://www.ashp.org/s_ashp/docs/files/discguide797-2008.pdf

Okeke, C. (2008, May 20). USP chapter <797> update on recent revisions. Retrieved from http://www.nabp.net/events/assets/UpdateonRevisions.pdf

USP797.org. (n.d.). Questions and answers on USP 797. Retrieved from http://www.usp797.org/Questions_and_Answers.htm

Automation Technician

LEARNING OBJECTIVES

Upon completion of this chapter, you will be able to

1. Understand automation technology terminology and concepts
2. Describe reasons for automation use in the hospital setting
3. Identify primary roles and responsibilities of an automation technician
4. Identify various reporting and maintenance functions for automation technology

KEY TERMS

Automated dispensing cabinet (ADC)
Automation
Biometrics
Blind count
Discrepancy
Diversion

Formulary
Inventory
Par level
Standard stock
Stock outs
Troubleshooting

INTRODUCTION

Automation is the use of technology to make tasks easier. Many areas in the pharmacy use automation to a greater or lesser degree, but don't necessarily refer to it as automation. When the term *automation* is commonly used, it is primarily in reference to medication dispensing technology. There are several major brands of dispensing technology, including Accudose, Meditrol, Suremed, Pyxis, and others. Although terms and format may differ, the purpose of these machines is nearly identical, and once familiar with one, it is much easier to learn another. This is similar to using either a Mac or a PC. They may have some differences in the look and navigation of their operating systems, but they are designed for the same purpose. A PC user can operate a Mac easier than someone who has never touched a computer at all.

MEDICATION DISPENSING OVERVIEW

Oral (PO) medications and other dosage forms not requiring IV room preparation are dispensed to nursing floors for administration, usually on a 24-hour basis. Before automation technology was available, this process was completed using the cart fill model. This model is still used in some facilities, sometimes in conjunction with automation. It is useful to understand the cart fill procedure in order to better see how automation has evolved from it. The principles of a cart fill are as follows:

- Each nursing unit has a mobile cart that has a drawer for each patient on the unit.
- This cart is brought to the pharmacy to be filled by a pharmacy technician.
- A report is generated from the pharmacy database daily that lists the drugs ordered for every patient in a given unit.
- A pharmacy technician determines the amount of medication needed for each patient for 24 hours of dosing.
- The technician proceeds to pull the medications needed from stock and places them in the corresponding drawer for each patient.
- Once verification has taken place, the filled cart is taken to the nursing unit.
- The nurses now have all medication ordered for their patients for the next 24 hours.

Another system that is used either independently or in conjunction with automation is what is known as patient-specific bins. These are bins located in the med room of nursing units that are designated for specific rooms for that unit. Instead of being on a cart, the technician brings patient doses to the med room and places them in the bin.

Automation technology speeds up these processes significantly by fundamentally changing how medication is dispensed. Instead of having drawers for specific patients, full of different medications, the medications are stored separately and accessed as needed for multiple patients. The foundation for this shift in filling methods is the invention of the **automated dispensing cabinet (ADC)**. This is the generic term used when not referring to a specific brand of machine (Grissinger, 2012).

An ADC takes the place of the medication cart used in cart fill procedures. Instead of being transported to a nursing unit on a daily basis, there is a stationary ADC located on each unit. When a nurse needs a specific medication for a patient, if it has been ordered and entered into the pharmacy database and is available in the ADC on that unit, the nurse can immediately remove it for administration. With cart fill, a newly ordered medication would have to be sent up from the pharmacy, increasing the time the nurse has to wait for it.

Anatomy of an ADC

An ADC can be likened to an automated teller machine (ATM) that dispenses drugs instead of money. This is because each machine is a locked unit that requires authorized access to get to medications. They are also controlled via a touch screen and keyboard interface. All have the ability to utilize barcode technology for increased medication safety and accuracy. Depending on the size of the nursing unit, machines can have auxiliary units that connect to the main ADC for increased storage capacity. **Figure 7-1** displays some of the components of a typical ADC:

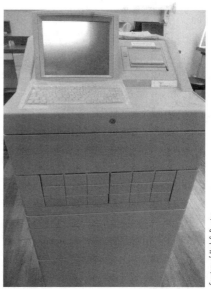

Courtesy of Mark G. Brunton.

FIGURE 7-1 Front view of an automated dispensing cabinet (ADC).

- *Touch screen interface:* Navigated by direct touch, this screen

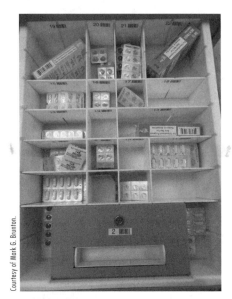

Courtesy of Mark G. Brunton.

FIGURE 7-2 A matrix drawer.

displays all of the functions available to a technician or nurse when accessing the machine.

- *Barcode scanner:* Used to verify correct medication during refill activities.
- *Receipt printer:* Prints receipts of user activity or report data upon request or based on preference settings.
- *Storage drawers:* Used to store medications for use as needed.

There are different types of storage drawers in terms of shape and function. This allows for the storage of many different sizes and types of medication, including controlled substances. The following different types can have other names and shapes, depending on brand:

- *Matrix drawer:* This drawer contains many pockets, each of which can hold a different medication (see **Figure 7-2**). It is highly customizable, with the ability to manually configure different size pockets depending on need. Controlled substances cannot be stored in this type of drawer, due to the open access nature of the pockets.

- *Return bin:* Located in matrix drawer configurations, this is a locked cabinet for nurses to return unused medication for retrieval by pharmacy staff.

- *Mini drawer:* This drawer opens only one set of pockets at a time, and can be configured to store either only one type of medication in the entire drawer or different types in each pocket (see **Figure 7-3**). When configured to store only one type,

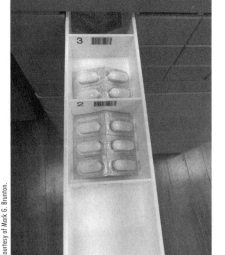

Courtesy of Mark G. Brunton.

FIGURE 7-3 A mini drawer.

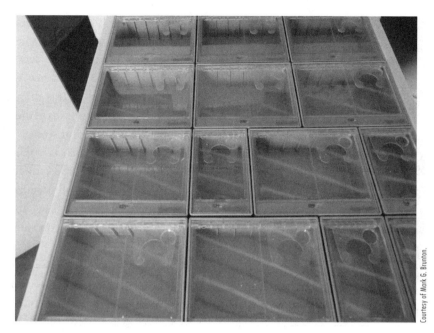

FIGURE 7-4 A sealed-pocket matrix.

this drawer is ideally suited for controlled-substance dispensing. It has the ability to open only one pocket at a time, which further limits access to the total amount of controlled substances available when dispensing.

- *Sealed-pocket matrix:* This is a combination of a matrix-style drawer with mini drawer control concepts (see **Figure 7-4**). The entire drawer opens, but each pocket is covered by a plastic lid. The ADC unlocks only one lid at a time. This allows for all types of medication to be stored in it, including both controlled and noncontrolled substances.

- *Carousel drawer:* The pockets in this drawer are wedge shaped, and are arranged in a circle (see **Figure 7-5**). It has a

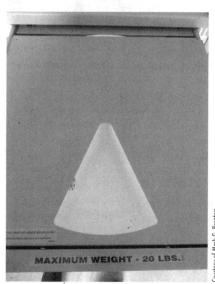

MAXIMUM WEIGHT - 20 LBS.

FIGURE 7-5 A carousel drawer.

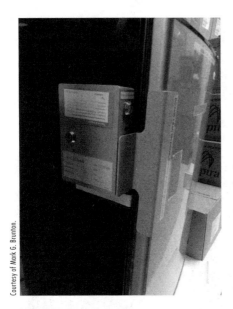

Courtesy of Mark G. Brunton.

FIGURE 7-6 A refrigerator manager.

metal lid that allows access to only one wedge at a time. The wedges rotate in order to provide access, much like a carousel, hence the name. The pockets of this drawer are deeper and larger than those of a matrix, allowing for storage of larger medications, such as oral liquid containers, unit dose syringes, and in some cases, small premixed IV bags. This drawer can hold both controlled and noncontrolled medications.

- *Refrigerator managers:* These electronically controlled locking mechanisms attach to a refrigerator located next to the ADC, turning it into a drawer for refrigerated meds (see **Figure 7-6**). It also has the ability to automatically record the internal temperature of the refrigerator, notifying the technician when it falls out of its prescribed range.

- *Tower drawers:* These are auxiliary units that consist of large shelves that can be configured with pockets for bigger items such as 1 L IV solutions (see **Figure 7-7**).

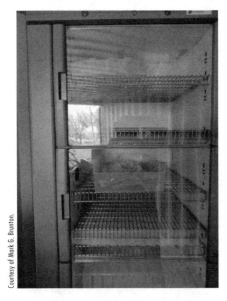

Courtesy of Mark G. Brunton.

FIGURE 7-7 A tower unit.

PRIMARY TECHNICIAN ADC ACTIVITIES

The main role of an automation technician is to resupply ADC cabinets with medications that are low in stock and to load medications in stations that do not have them. This activity can take up a significant portion of the daily workflow. A medium-sized hospital can have from 35 to 40 ADC cabinets that have to be refilled. Certain concepts are essential to this process, and are discussed in the following sections.

TIPS AND TRICKS
Manuals: The Best Thing You've Never Read

If you ask the majority of people you know if they have read the manual for a major appliance or device they have purchased, the results are almost universally no.

I would classify myself in the smaller group of people who actually say, "Yes," as well as, "I have a file folder for all my manuals." I love reading manuals. I want to know every possible little detail about whatever TV I am using, phone I am calling on, or video game I am about to play. This mindset is not something to be overlooked in the pharmacy workplace.

There is always a manual available for the technology used in the pharmacy. It is almost guaranteed that if you look around the main console of the ADC system, for example, you will find the manual on how to operate it. It is almost a sure bet that it is dusty. This is because nobody bothers to read the manual. When the system was first implemented, the company most likely sent out trainers to orient staff, and from then on training was done from one technician to another, passed down like the oral history of a village.

By actually reading the manual, a technician will probably find many useful features and options that no one else in the department knows about. These features and options can make your daily activities quicker and easier or affect system-level options that can streamline the entire department. This knowledge helps make you less dispensable to the department, and demonstrates a willingness to improve a skill set without prompting. That sets you apart from the pack. So don't hesitate to read the manual. Clichéd as it sounds, knowledge is power.

Batch Filling

Batch filling is similar in structure to an IV batch fill. The technician generates reports for each ADC in the hospital. These refill reports list the medications that are below par level in each ADC. A **par level** is the minimum and maximum amount of a drug that should be loaded into a given machine. This level can be adjusted depending on need or lack thereof. An example of a par level would be for Tylenol in a given unit, with a minimum (min) of 4 and a maximum (max) of 10. This means that if the number of Tylenol caplets in that machine drops below 4, it will show up as an item on the refill report. This level would then be refilled to the maximum of 10 caplets.

The technician would then begin to pull the meds on the report. The term *pull* refers to the fact that most hospital pharmacies store their medications on shelves in narrow plastic bins, and these bins are pulled off of the shelf to get to the medications. The number of each medication to be pulled is determined by the max level listed on the refill report. Using the previous example, if the number of Tylenol located in the machine is 3, and the max is 10, then the refill amount pulled would be 7. Note, however, that unit dose medications commonly are packaged in multiples of 10. It is not uncommon to pull in multiples of 10 for efficiency, as long as the drawer or pocket can accommodate the amount over the max. For example, if a par level was 20 and there were only 2 left, the most accurate refill amount would be 18. But it would probably be easier to pull two packages of 10 and fill them.

The pulled medications are then either placed in plastic baggies or rubber banded together, and arranged on the fill counter for pharmacist verification. Organized placement of medications is recommended for speedier verification. This placement is commonly in columns starting at the top left of the check counter and moving to the right, in the same order as the beginning of the report (**Figure 7-8**).

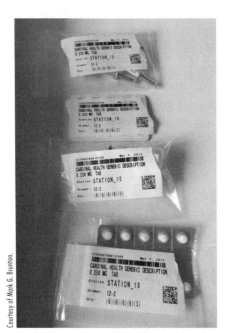

Courtesy of Mark G. Brunton.

FIGURE 7-8 Medications awaiting verification for ADC fill.

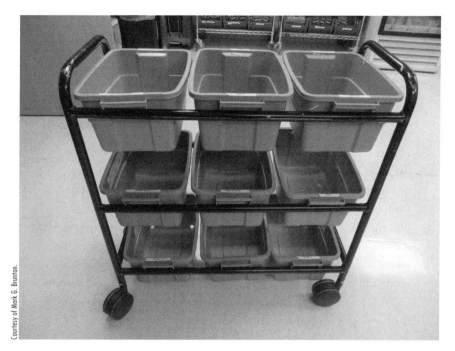

Courtesy of Mark G. Brunton.

FIGURE 7-9 An example of a delivery cart used to bring medications to nursing units.

Once verified, the medications are stored in locations for each unit and are then ready for transport to their respective ADCs for refill activities (**Figure 7-9**).

IN THE FIELD
Tech Check Tech

The idea for a tech check tech has been around for several years, but only recently has it begun to rise in prominence, mainly in the hospital setting. The concept behind the term is that certain activities legally can be verified by another technician rather than a pharmacist. Its increasing use can be attributed to many factors, such as the increasing education of technicians via formalized training and national certification, and the desire for pharmacists to spend more time performing clinical functions.

Although the traditional pattern of thinking is that a pharmacist must personally check every medication that leaves the pharmacy, there are specific points to consider in favor of tech check tech. IV and ADC batch refill activities do not result in the medication being dispensed directly to a patient; rather, these batches are being delivered to a nursing unit's medication room or ADC. It is the nurse who is responsible for the administration of the medication. The theory is that the technician is only moving stock from one area of the facility to another. When a technician moves a medication from one shelf to another in the pharmacy, they do not need a pharmacist to come and sign off on it, so why would it be necessary if it is only being moved to another room in the hospital? With the use of barcodes to increase accuracy, this practice is being looked at more and more favorably. So do not be surprised if you are asked by another technician to check their batch refill before it is delivered to the nursing unit (**Figure 7-10**).

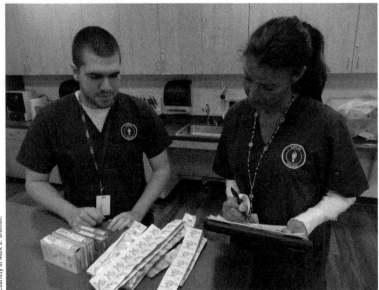

Courtesy of Mark G. Brunton.

FIGURE 7-10 Tech check tech is being utilized more often in today's hospital settings.

Stock Outs

The main console automatically prints notifications when certain events take place with the ADCs in the facility. One of these notifications deals with **stock outs**. A stock out is when a medication is completely empty in a given ADC. These occur even if the medication was on the batch fill report. It may have been below par when the batch refill report was generated, but then the remaining medication was used before the batch fill was actually delivered. This scenario can be thought of as if when driving a vehicle, the gasoline gauge showed the tank was almost empty, but then the car ran completely out before actually getting to a gas station. This notification should be attended to in a timely fashion.

When a stock out notification is generated, the technician has two options:

1. If the medication is already in the batch refill, and delivery is imminent, the notice can be disregarded because the medication will soon be refilled.
2. If the medication was not on the refill list, or the delivery of the batch will not occur relatively soon, the medication may be delivered separate from the batch.

Ordered Medication Not Loaded

This notification is generated when a medication needs to be *loaded* into an ADC. There is a difference between a refill and a load. Each ADC in a given hospital does not have the exact same medications loaded in them. An ADC in an intensive care unit (ICU) will have medications that are not stored in an ADC on a different, less critical care floor, for example. When a patient has an order for a medication that is not stored in the ADC where they are located, a med not loaded notification is generated. This tells the technician what drug is needed and which ADC it must be put into for the nurse to be able to access it.

The technician must do the following in order to handle this notification:

1. Determine par levels to be set for the given medication. This is done by analyzing the sig, or instructions for use, of the order and calculating the appropriate amount needed to satisfy at least 24 hours' worth of dosing. For example, if the order was for metformin 500 mg tabs twice daily, the minimum quantity that would need to be loaded would be two tablets. It is more common to load a 72-hour supply.
2. Identify available storage space in the necessary ADC for placement of the new medication.

3. Pull the medication requested in the pharmacy.

4. Have the medication verified for accuracy.

5. Load the medication into the ADC cabinet.

Real Estate

There are generally more medications that can be loaded than available space in a given ADC unit. The process of identifying an available pocket to load a new medication can at times be challenging. This is like having prime real estate. It is always in demand, and competition for space can be fierce. In the case of an ADC, if the machine is full, the technician must identify a medication that is already loaded but has not been used in a certain amount of time. This indicates that it would be safe to remove that medication from the unit in order to make room for the new ordered medication. This information can be searched for in the main console.

Return Bin Operations

There are times when a nurse will withdraw a medication from an ADC for administration, but for one reason or another end up not giving it to the patient. This can occur if the patient is transferred or is taken for a procedure, for example. In these cases a nurse can go back to the ADC and return the medication. The medication is returned through a locked drop box. These actions credit the medication back to the patient, saving them unnecessary charges. They also allow the pharmacy to return the unused medication to stock.

When a technician is refilling an ADC, they may also empty the return bin. When this function is accessed at the station, the drawer containing the return bin will open. The technician would then proceed to unlock the bin and remove the medications from within. The display on the ADC will list the items that should be in the return bin. The technician must verify that there are no missing medications, especially controlled substances. If there is a difference between what is physically in the return bin versus what is listed on the display, the technician must log the discrepancy.

SECONDARY TECHNICIAN ACTIVITIES

There are additional features and functions of ADC technology besides medication dispensing. A pharmacy technician can perform additional activities and tasks that utilize these features. These activities are not limited to only the automation technician. Other positions may need to perform some of these tasks, and other times a supervisor may also be involved.

Reports

Every transaction or interaction that occurs with an ADC is recorded and sent to the main console. This wealth of data can be used to analyze many different aspects of medication use within the hospital. There are several premade reports that can be generated from the main console, but custom reports can also be created. The following are examples of the different types of reports that can be generated.

Loaded Medications Not Ordered

This report can be used to better manage the limited real estate of pockets available for loading new medications. It lists the medications in a particular machine that are not ordered for any patient on that floor or unit. The report also often states the last time the medication was ordered for a patient on said floor. This is used to determine whether it is a good idea to unload that medication to make room for other needed medications. If the medication was ordered for a patient less than a week prior, it may not be a good candidate for unloading. One that hasn't been ordered for several months would be a better option. The only exception to this process would be standard stock items. **Standard stock** medications are a group of medications that should never be unloaded from a station, regardless of whether a patient currently has an order for them. These may be life-saving drugs, or drugs that have been determined to be essential in each machine. Extra Strength Tylenol, for example, is often loaded into every ADC in a hospital, and is never unloaded. *Someone* is going to have an order for it at some point. Standard stock items are usually clearly identified in any reports generated.

A technician can generate a loaded medications not ordered report, analyze it, and then proceed to remove selected medications from different ADC cabinets and return them to the pharmacy. This creates available pockets for any newly ordered medications that need to be loaded.

Medication Search

This report is created to list all of the locations where a particular medication is loaded. For example, a search could be done for Levaquin 500 mg tablets. The report would list every machine that has this drug loaded, and also how many tablets are physically present in each machine. This can be useful when a particular medication is on back order or not available due to a shortage from the manufacturer. Excess and unused stock can be consolidated for use in critical areas or as needed.

Another version of the search report can be generated to show the access history of a particular medication. A technician could run an access report for Oxycontin 10 mg tablets. The report would show every transaction for that particular medication within the specified time frame. This would include every nurse who accessed it, when they accessed it, and how much they accessed. It could also show every technician who filled, inventoried, loaded, or unloaded it as well. This could be run for a particular ADC unit or hospital-wide. The report can be configured for a specified time or date range as well.

These data can be used to analyze usage, and also to track potential diversion. **Diversion** is the term used in pharmacy for theft. This theft is almost always of controlled substances, but is not limited to it. By analyzing access to high-risk items, patterns can be found that may be indications of diversion. There are built-in analytical programs that can scan for these patterns automatically and warn of potential diversions within the hospital.

Access

All employees of the hospital who use an ADC must be given access to the system. Technicians, nurses, anesthesiologists, and others must have a secure means of logging into the system. The standard method is to be assigned a login ID and password. The current trend is to use biometrics rather than a password for access. **Biometrics** refers to technology that analyzes unique biological characteristics for identity verification. In popular movies, this can be seen as a retinal scanner of the eye for entry into a secure location (see **Figure 7-11**).

For ADC technology, the biometric most often used for access is a fingerprint. For an employee to access an ADC, they would enter their login and place a designated fingertip on a laser scanner mounted to the machine (see **Figure 7-12**). To date, this method is the most secure means of identification for ADC technology. Login IDs and passwords can be stolen; it is much more difficult to fake a user's fingerprint.

Access can vary according to position as well. Depending on an employee's role in the hospital, their level of access will vary. This means that a pharmacy technician will have the ability to do certain activities with an ADC that a nurse will not, and vice versa.

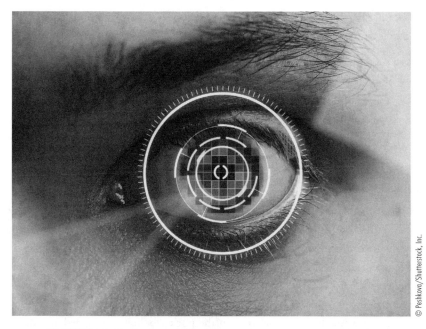

FIGURE 7-11 Biometric identification systems increase security for access to medications.

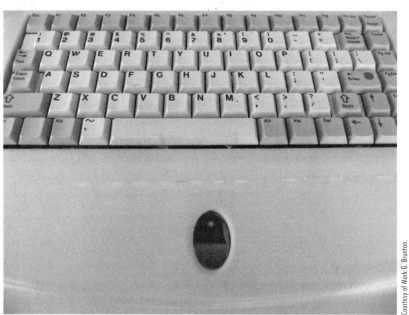

FIGURE 7-12 Biometric fingerprint scanner.

A pharmacy technician may have control over access functions that include the following:

- Assigning access to new users
- Resetting access for employees
- Changing the level of access for employees when necessary
- Deleting user profiles for employees who were terminated, transferred, or have left the employment of the facility

Inventory

The **inventory** is the actual number of medications on hand in a given ADC or in the entire hospital. Taking an inventory of an ADC involves physically counting the medications stored in it. This can be done for one particular medication or many. The ADC keeps a running inventory automatically, which is verified whenever a particular medication is accessed. This count can be inaccurate due to human error, however. There are two settings for inventory activities. The general setting is for the machine to open the pocket being inventoried and display the count of doses that *should* be physically present. The technician would then count the medication in the pocket and verify its accuracy. The other setting is what is known as a **blind count.** This is always used for controlled substances, high-cost medications, or others at risk for diversion. It differs from the standard setting in that when the pocket opens for the inventory, the presumed number is *not* displayed. The technician must type in the number physically in the pocket after counting them. The ADC then compares this number with what it thinks *should* be in there based on prior access. If there is a difference or error, the user is allowed one additional opportunity to input a count. This is in case the previous entry was entered in error due to an incorrect key press or the user miscounted. If the number is still inconsistent, a **discrepancy** is created. A discrepancy is an alert generated when a controlled substance or other monitored drug is unaccounted for. This alert is recorded in the system and must be cleared by explaining the nature of the error and accounting for the missing medication.

Formulary Maintenance

A **formulary** is a list of medications. This could refer to the hospital formulary, which is all of the medications approved for use in the facility. When referred to in connection with automation, it is the list of medications programmed into the main console database.

As new medications become available, or if multiple manufacturers for the same drug are used, this information must be updated in the system. This is especially true with bar code technology. Formulary maintenance should be reserved for technicians who have had experience with the system, or those with specific training.

Troubleshooting, Repair, and Maintenance

Automation technology brings with it many benefits: efficiency, accuracy, and financial savings, to name a few. It also creates new areas of responsibility in terms of managing it. All technology has the potential for bugs, glitches, and malfunctions that have to be addressed. It also has new procedures involved with maintenance and upkeep. This is almost exclusively the domain of the pharmacy technician.

Troubleshooting

One of the types of calls from nursing to pharmacy deals with utilizing ADC technology. Challenges can vary from a nurse not being able to remove a particular medication to there being a physical malfunction with the ADC itself. Depending on the particular technology used and setup in a given facility, there will be many situations to deal with. Only practice and experience will allow you to handle all of them. The process used is known as **troubleshooting**. This is a systematic approach to solving problems quickly and efficiently.

If you have read a manual to solve a malfunction or looked at the help file for a particular piece of software, you have most likely seen a written troubleshooting guide. It consists of a list of questions or criteria used to determine the most likely problem and solution for it. This same idea is applied regarding ADC problems. By asking specific questions, you can narrow down the list of potential problems and identify the correct course of action. These questions may be answered by direct communication with nursing staff, or they may require more research into the system by the technician. For ADC technology, the most common problem that is dealt with is when a nurse cannot get a needed medication out of the machine. Determining why the medication is inaccessible is the next step. When troubleshooting, you might ask some of the following questions:

- Is the medication loaded in that particular unit?
- Is the medication out of stock?
- Is the medication order for that particular patient entered into the patient's profile yet?
- Is the drawer where the medication is loaded inaccessible due to a mechanical malfunction?

There may be more questions or different ones, depending on the type of ADC technology in use. Don't forget that the console manual will most likely have a written troubleshooting guide in it. Use it to familiarize yourself with the most common problems encountered and their possible solutions.

Repair

How many times has your car broken down or computer frozen? The answer for most of us is at least once, if not multiple times. ADC technology consists of many electronic and mechanical components. These components can and do break from time to time. Software may crash or freeze and drawers may break or jam. These problems are often beyond the scope or expertise of a pharmacy technician. In those situations, the technician must notify the service technician that works for the ADC company to come out and service the machine.

The service number is generally posted somewhere in the department. When calling, the technician would identify the following pieces of information to the service technician:

- His/her name and the name of the facility
- The nature of the malfunction or service required

When talking to the service department, it is recommended to ask for the projected time of arrival by service personnel. This is useful for follow-up activities. The technician should then communicate with coworkers and staff as to the nature of the problem and the expected turnaround time involved. If it is going to be several hours or more, the technician should identify alternative means for nursing to receive the necessary medication, such as generating a label and sending up a unit dose from the main pharmacy.

TIPS AND TRICKS
Making Friends with Your Service Technician

It is, of course, good to be friendly and courteous with everyone you work with, if possible. It is very good to make friends with your ADC service technician as well (**Figure 7-13**). This doesn't mean you have to hang out with or call him or her on the phone. Merely knowing his or her name and making polite and friendly conversation is enough.

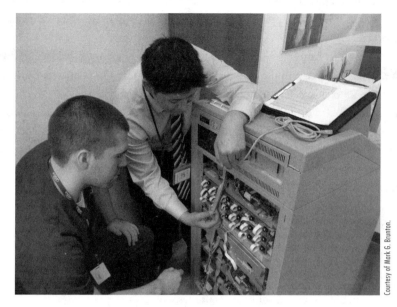

FIGURE 7-13 Depiction of a good relationship with a service technician.

If a service technician needs to work on a machine on a nursing unit, it is customary for a pharmacy technician to accompany them, in order to be responsible for any medications that will be accessed during the repair procedure. Although they are working on the machine, this is an excellent time to ask about the nature of what they are working on. Being curious about the technology you work with is a good trait to have. Sometimes a pharmacy technician can learn enough to turn some issues that require a service call into something they can fix on their own. If not, they will at least be able to more effectively communicate technical problems if they have to call the service technician again.

Maintenance

Just like an automobile, regular maintenance of ADC units will prevent more severe problems from occurring down the road. There are many areas of maintenance, both mechanically and electronically. Many times the recommended maintenance activities are overlooked, and are done sporadically or not at all. This is an excellent area to become proficient in and show extra value to the department.

One of the easiest procedures to complete is to keep the drawers in the machines clean. An ampule may break or an oral liquid dose cup may leak while stored in a pocket. Many staff and employees may not take the time to clean up the spilled medication. This can then lead to the drawer becoming sticky, leaking onto electrical components, and just being plain messy. Foam inserts and other options are available to also help minimize breakage of medication. It is also beneficial to remove medications in machines that have not been used in a certain amount of time. This will help alleviate the previously mentioned real estate challenge, and provide available pockets for newly ordered medications (Institute for Safe Medication Practices, 2008).

Electronically, it is good to periodically review the formulary in the main console in order to delete items that are no longer used in the facility. This is similar to weeding out dead plants in a garden. This helps prevent selection errors when loading medications and for other activities.

The manual for the system is again a terrific resource for maintenance suggestions and schedules. This is also another area of inquiry for the service technician when they come to visit. A service technician in any discipline can appreciate those who take care of the machinery they have to service, because it makes their job easier and prevents many problems before they even occur.

SUMMARY

Automated dispensing technology is a common element in many hospital pharmacies. Familiarity with the concepts of how they function and their use allows a pharmacy technician to learn different systems more quickly. A technician who strives to learn every aspect of the technology they have to deal with on a daily basis will be a valuable asset to the department.

Technology is continually improving and hospitals are transitioning into a fully electronic environment. This includes bedside bar code scanning technology, electronic health records and medical administration records, and even computerized physician order entry. A technician in a hospital setting would do well to always be on the leading edge of the technology they will interact with. It is always better to be in a position to help others transition rather than being the one who needs to be helped. This is not a quality that will be necessarily trained or expected, and therefore is memorable when used. Besides all of these benefits, knowing how ADC technology works allows you to work more efficiently, no matter what position is being covered in the department.

REVIEW QUESTIONS

1. What method of medication dispensing activities was replaced by the advent of automation in the health system setting?
2. Describe how an ADC improves the medication dispensing process over older methods.
3. What kinds of storage areas can exist in an ADC, and how are they used?
4. Where can controlled substances be stored in an ADC?
5. Describe the steps in a batch fill for an ADC.
6. What are par levels, and how do they affect ADC dispensing functions?
7. Give some examples of standard stock medications.
8. What does diversion mean? What are a technician's responsibilities when diversion is suspected?
9. Define biometrics and its role in ADC technology.
10. What are some maintenance activities that a pharmacy technician can perform on ADCs?

REFERENCES

Grissinger, M. (2012). Safeguards for using and designing automated dispensing cabinets. *Pharmacy and Therapeutics, 37*(9), 490–491. Retrieved from http://www.ncbi.nlm.nih.gov/pmc/articles/PMC3462599/

Institute for Safe Medication Practices (ISMP). (2008). Guidance on the interdisciplinary safe use of automated dispensing cabinets. Retrieved from http://www.ismp.org/tools/guidelines/ADC_Guidelines_final.pdf

CHAPTER 8

Specialty Roles and Duties

LEARNING OBJECTIVES

Upon completion of this chapter, you will be able to

1. Define the roles and responsibilities for specialty technician positions in a hospital pharmacy
2. Understand the training or experience required for specialty positions
3. Describe how specialty roles interact with other positions in hospital pharmacy

KEY TERMS

DEA 222 form

Decentralized pharmacy

Discrepancy

Diversion

Fast mover

Medication reconciliation

Narcotic log sheet

Recall

Satellite pharmacy

Scheduled drug

Want list

INTRODUCTION

Some positions in hospital pharmacy are classified as "specialty" or "advanced." These positions require more experience and training and are not universal to all hospital pharmacies. This can be due to the size or budget of a given facility. If these positions do not exist in the format described, the tasks laid out still typically exist in some fashion, but may be assigned to other positions.

PURCHASING AGENT

The common nickname for the purchasing agent is the buyer. This position is responsible for the acquisition of all medication used in a hospital pharmacy. The buyer's daily responsibilities can include:

- Identifying medications that need to be purchased
- Placing orders for medication to wholesalers or distributors
- Operating within the allotted budget for purchases
- Managing medication recalls and shortages

Creating the Order

Buyers will typically "walk the shelves," visually inspecting the stock of medications in a pharmacy. Medications that are low in stock, or are known to be fast movers, are then placed on the order. **Fast movers** are certain medications that are used heavily in a given facility. These drugs are ordered more often and in larger quantities than other pharmacy stock.

Buyers utilize a handheld scanner device in order to compile the order (see **Figure 8-1**). Adding medications to the order involves scanning the barcode for that particular medication and indicating the quantity to be ordered. The device then uploads the information to the purchasing software on the buyer's computer. Medication orders are placed on a daily basis.

© Benjamin Haas/Shutterstock, Inc.

FIGURE 8-1 A purchasing agent adding medications to an order.

Placing the Order

Once the order has been compiled and uploaded to the buyer's computer, a new order can be placed. It is submitted electronically. The buyer keeps track of all purchase order numbers, invoices, and billing paperwork that are associated with the order. Good communication between pharmacy staff and the buyer is essential to ensure an adequate stock of required drugs. With so many different drugs in a pharmacy, the buyer is unable to identify every medication that needs to be ordered daily. They rely on other staff, most often the central, IV, and automation technicians, to communicate any unanticipated drug use. A common way to communicate these needs is with a want list. The **want list** is a sheet on which pharmacy staff can write down items for the buyer to order. Utilization of this list by technicians is essential to maintain adequate levels of drugs in the pharmacy. When a drug is out of stock, technicians have been known to ask a buyer, "Why didn't (*name of drug*) come in?" to which many a buyer has responded, "Did you put it on the want list?" The reply is generally a sheepish, "No."

Budgets

The buyer reports to the director of pharmacy (DOP) or assistant DOP regarding budget constraints and drug availability. If they are given a specific monthly budget, the buyer will try to remain within that budget while placing orders. If a medication order will go over budget, the buyer must be prepared to justify the additional costs.

Drug Recalls and Shortages

Recurring issues with drug manufacturers are the recalls and shortages of various medications. A **recall** is when a specific lot of medication is asked to be returned to the manufacturer. When this occurs, it is the buyer's responsibility to determine if any of the recalled medication is in the facility. If so, they coordinate retrieval and return shipping of the medication.

If there is a shortage of a medication, the buyer will try to locate alternative sources of the medication based on need in the facility. They will also notify pharmacy staff of any shortages that would affect medication availability. Many times alternative medications can be used in place of the unavailable one. Buyers receive notices of drug recalls and backorders on a weekly basis.

Purchasing Agent Summary

A buyer is usually a technician who has had at least 1 year or more of experience in hospital pharmacy. Most are promoted from within, because the technician already has experience with the drug use in that particular facility. The technology utilized includes computerized ordering software and handheld barcode scanning devices. There is usually one buyer per hospital pharmacy, with a second technician trained in their duties for coverage during either weekends or vacation. There are also positions for regional buyers, who manage several buyers in a network of hospitals.

SATELLITE TECHNICIAN

Larger hospitals are more likely to use the decentralized pharmacy model for operations. A **decentralized pharmacy** is composed of a main pharmacy and several smaller pharmacies located throughout the facility. These smaller pharmacies are referred to as **satellite pharmacies**. These satellites are responsible for certain nursing units or patient care areas. A satellite allows a pharmacist and technician to interact with nursing more directly in patient medication therapy and clinical functions. They are able to communicate face-to-face with nursing staff and doctors on a daily basis. This relieves the workload on the main pharmacy department.

The duties of a satellite technician are similar to those of a central technician. Medication dispensing and telephone answering duties are performed in the satellite location. Additional responsibilities may include:

- Medication order entry
- Clinical information gathering for pharmacist review
- Limited IV preparation

Medication Order Entry

A satellite technician may have the responsibility of entering medication orders into the computer for the unit their satellite is responsible for. This process of order entry follows the same pattern as for medication dispensing activities:

1. The technician enters the order into the computer database.
2. A pharmacist verifies the completeness and accuracy of the entry.
3. The medication order is processed and dispensed.

Clinical Information Gathering

The benefit of having a satellite pharmacy is that there are a dedicated pharmacist and technician for certain areas. In this model, the pharmacist has more expanded roles in the realm of medication therapy management. One activity, for example, is that a pharmacist may review the patients in their area to determine IV to PO conversion status. They would research the feasibility of changing a given patient's medications from IV formulations to oral versions in order to save money and increase convenience for the patient.

A satellite technician may help in this and other activities by assisting in gathering information about selected patients for the pharmacist. This might include screening patient profiles, communicating with nursing staff, and finding information in the patient's chart.

Limited IV Preparations

If there is a glovebox, or barrier isolator, in the satellite pharmacy, a technician is able to compound preparations for use on the nursing unit. They may provide first doses and stat doses, and assist in other preparations as required. It is unlikely that there would be a full IV compounding room dedicated to a satellite pharmacy in any but the largest and most affluent hospital settings.

Satellite Technician Summary

Different areas that may have satellite pharmacies include the surgery department, emergency room, medical floors, and intensive care units. The requirements for this position are the same as for a central technician. Strong customer service skills and a positive attitude are especially important for a technician in this position, as well as the ability to work unsupervised. This is common if the pharmacist is out on the nursing unit communicating with doctors and nurses about patient care.

CONTROLLED SUBSTANCE TECHNICIAN

The Controlled Substances Act of 1970 created the laws and regulations that govern all drugs that have the potential for abuse. As a result, these controlled substances, also known as **scheduled drugs**, must be kept secured in the hospital setting. Every tablet, patch, and even milliliter of a controlled substance must be accounted for. The nursing department is also required to keep accurate records upon administration. Many hospital pharmacies have a technician position dedicated to the handling of controlled substances. The controlled substance technician's duties may include:

- Ordering controlled substances from the manufacturer
- Dispensing and record keeping of controlled substances
- Discrepancy resolution
- Diversion tracking

Ordering Controlled Substances

The procedures for ordering controlled substances are very specific. A **DEA 222 form** is the legal document required by the Drug Enforcement Administration to place orders for CII medications (see **Figure 8-2**). *CII* stands for controlled substance Class II. There are also classifications III through V. The lower the

BLANK DEA FORM-222
U.S. OFFICIAL ORDER FORM - SCHEDULES I & II

See Reverse of PURCHASER'S Copy of Instructions		No order form may be issued for Schedule I and II substances unless a completed application form has been received, (21 CFR 1305.04).			OMB APPROVAL No. 1117-0010
TO: *(Name of Supplier)*			STREET ADDRESS		
CITY and STATE		DATE	**TO BE FILLED IN BY SUPPLIER**		
			SUPPLIERS DEA REGISTRATION No.		

L I N E No	No. of Packages	Size of Package	TO BE FILLED IN BY PURCHASER — Name of Item	National Drug Code	Packages Shipped	Date Shipped
1						
2						
3						
4						
5						
6						
7						
8						
9						
10						

◀ **LAST LINE COMPLETED** *(MUST BE 10 OR LESS)* SIGNATURE OR PURCHASER OR ATTORNEY OR AGENT

Date Issued	DEA Registration No.	Name and Address of Registrant
Schedules		
Registered as a	No. of this Order Form	

DEA Form-222 (Oct. 1992)

U.S. OFFICIAL ORDER FORMS - SCHEDULES I & II
DRUG ENFORCEMENT ADMINISTRATION
SUPPLIER'S Copy 1

Courtesy of U.S. Drug Enforcement Administration, U.S. Department of Justice.

Note: The graphic illustrated above is only a depiction of the DEA Form-222. It is not intended to be used as an actual order form.

FIGURE 8-2 A DEA 222 form.

number is, the higher the potential for abuse of the medication. CII medications are therefore the strongest of the controlled substances. CIII–CV medications can be ordered by the buyer or other designated personnel with the regular medication order. Mistakes are not allowed on 222 forms. If there is an error, the technician is required to void it and use a new form. Crossing out an error or using white-out is prohibited. The form must be filled out in ink, not pencil. There are now versions of the 222 form that are filled out on a computer and transmitted electronically. These electronic 222 forms greatly increase the accuracy and efficiency of CII ordering.

Dispensing and Record Keeping

All controlled substances are stored in a secure location in the pharmacy. A **narcotic log sheet** is a paper form that is used to keep track of these drugs. Every time the quantity of these drugs changes, it is recorded in the log book. These changes occur from removals for dispensing, additions to stock, returns, and any wasted medication (see **Figure 8-3**).

Many hospitals have utilized automated dispensing cabinet (ADC) technology to keep accurate counts of their controlled substances. There are specialized ADC devices that can be located in the pharmacy and used to store the department's scheduled drugs (see **Figure 8-4**). In order to dispense them to other areas of the facility, a technician would log in and withdraw them in much the same way nurses remove medications on the floor for their patients.

Discrepancies

A **discrepancy** is an error between the narcotic log and the physical inventory of a medication. This means that there could be more actual stock than what is listed in the log. Of greater concern is when there is less physical stock than is recorded. This error can occur within the pharmacy as well as on the nursing unit. The reasons for discrepancies vary. Often the cause is a minor math error when adding or subtracting quantities from the log book. It is the responsibility of the narcotic technician to investigate discrepancies in the log book and discover the cause of them. Once the explanation for the discrepancy has been found, the technician can properly document the error.

Typically, nursing is responsible for documenting and clearing any discrepancies created by their department. It is also the responsibility of the controlled substance technician to follow up and make inquiries if this task is not

NARCOTIC & CONTROLLED DRUG ACCOUNTABILITY GUIDELINES

NARCOTICS AND CONTROLLED DRUGS
PERPETUAL INVENTORY FORM

DRUG NAME & STRENGTH: _____   DOSAGE FORM: _____

DATE: _____

PURCHASES			PRESCRIPTIONS			STARTING INVENTORY OR BALANCE FORWARD	PHARMACIST'S SIGNATURE	
Invoice #	Date Received	Quantity Received	Rx Number	Date Filled	Quantity Dispensed	Current Inventory		

These records must be kept for a minimum of 2 years.

FIGURE 8-3 Controlled substances log sheet.

completed within the specified time limit. This is usually by the end of a nurse's shift.

Diversion Tracking

Diversion is the term used for theft in the pharmacy. If a drug is being misappropriated for someone other than its intended recipient, and if it is being used for something other than its intended function, it is being diverted. Narcotics are the main class of drugs that are diverted, but by no means are they the only ones. Anyone in the healthcare team that has access

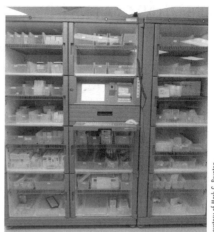

FIGURE 8-4 A CII safe.

to narcotics has the ability to divert them. This could be a technician, pharmacist, nurse, or doctor. An unusual number of discrepancies is one potential indicator of diversion taking place (O'Neal, 2011). The responsibility for investigating potential diversion can be assigned to the controlled substance technician, but can also be assigned to a technician supervisor or pharmacist. The technician will be trained in the specific policies and procedures to follow if diversion is suspected, as outlined in the facility. A controlled substance technician will develop an awareness of the standard usage and quantity of the narcotics that they are responsible for. This awareness can help to alert the technician if there is a pattern that deviates from that standard. A respected doctor and speaker at a national convention stated, "If you don't have a problem with diversion in your facility, then you aren't looking hard enough" (Siegel, 2010). This statement is truer than many realize. An alert controlled substance technician can help to minimize these events and identify them if they are occurring, so that appropriate action can be taken.

Controlled Substance Technician Summary

A controlled substance technician is a highly trusted position, because the risk of diversion is so high. This role involves interacting with nurses, doctors, and anesthesiologists in order to resolve discrepancies. In order to be effective at diversion tracking, the ability to spot patterns and anomalies in dispensing volume is required.

TECHNICIAN SUPERVISOR

Every pharmacist is technically a supervisor of technicians, and can assign tasks and duties as necessary. Many pharmacies also employ a technician to manage most of the supervisory duties for their technician staff. These duties may include:

- Weekly scheduling of positions for pharmacy staff
- Preparation and maintenance of employee files
- Continuing education completion monitoring
- Performance evaluations and disciplinary duties
- Hiring and termination duties

Many additional responsibilities can be assigned to this position; as a result, the technician supervisor may not perform regular technician functions in busier hospitals. In other situations, a technician supervisor may have these responsibilities *in addition* to working regular shifts and job duties. Experience in the field is a must, with training in management techniques being highly useful.

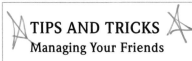

TIPS AND TRICKS
Managing Your Friends

There are many resources available for those who want to learn how to manage and lead employees better. Books, websites, and seminars abound with material on how to be the best manager you can be. There are also many different theories and styles of management to choose from. The author encourages any technician who is interested in management to seek out these resources and select or study what seems to be the best fit, if not utilizing elements from many. One thing that almost every manager can agree on, however, is this principle:

If one has even the slightest urge to go into management at a given facility, that person must *never* become close with those they could potentially manage, because it will be next to impossible to discipline that subordinate if necessary, and there is great potential for the close friend to take advantage of that friendship, *even unintentionally*. Also realize that even if that were not to happen, others in the department could still perceive favoritism. This is not to say you cannot be friend*ly*, but a distance in personal lives and friend*ship* must be avoided or minimized in order to succeed as a manager. The only alternative would be to move into a supervisory position at *another* facility.

AUTOMATION MANAGER

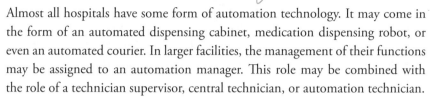

Almost all hospitals have some form of automation technology. It may come in the form of an automated dispensing cabinet, medication dispensing robot, or even an automated courier. In larger facilities, the management of their functions may be assigned to an automation manager. This role may be combined with the role of a technician supervisor, central technician, or automation technician.

Their duties may include:

- Troubleshooting and maintenance
- Communication with device representatives and service technicians
- Space allocation
- User access

In large hospitals that have dozens of ADC cabinets, the roles listed may not be able to be completed by the automation technician alone. The majority of their time would be spent just trying to get all of the machines refilled for the day. This is when an automation manager role can be created, in order to keep these ancillary tasks from piling up due to their secondary nature.

A technician in this position has extensive experience with the particular automation used at the facility. This role is semiautonomous, and the ability to work effectively unsupervised is required. Technicians in this role may have the opportunity to move into roles working for the manufacturers of the automation technology they manage, as service technicians, representatives, and applications specialists. Although these career paths are potentially open to anyone with the proper qualifications, automation managers tend to have a higher chance and more connections for employment in this arena.

MEDICATION RECONCILIATION TECHNICIAN

This role is one of the newest to be implemented in the hospital for technicians. **Medication reconciliation** is the process by which a patient being admitted to the hospital lists all of the medications they are currently taking. This list is then compared to any medication orders that are written by the hospital physician upon admission. This comparison checks for duplication of therapy, missing medication, and contraindications. This information was originally gathered by nursing staff. A technician utilized in this task is more cost effective and frees up both the pharmacist and nurse for other duties that utilize their clinical training. It is a prime example of the expansion of pharmacy technician duties. This role is unique in its responsibilities. They may include:

- Interacting with emergency department and admissions staff
- Face-to-face interaction with newly admitted patients and family members
- Communication with retail pharmacies or family practice physicians
- Data input

This position generally operates directly out of the emergency or admissions departments. Specialized training is required on the methods of communication with patients and their family members. Empathy and excellent communication skills are required as well (**Figure 8-5**). A broad knowledge of drug names and classifications is also very useful in this position.

Community setting technicians are often sought out to be employed as medication reconciliation techs. This is due to the retail technician's abundant experience communicating with doctors and patients directly (Barreto, Ebert, Maier, & Wooton, 2008).

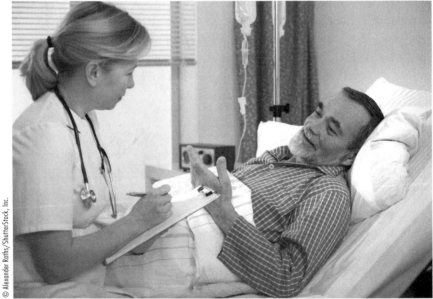

© Alexander Raths/ShutterStock, Inc.

FIGURE 8-5 Medication reconciliation requires good communication skills.

SUMMARY

There are many different and specialized areas of technician practice that exist for advancement. Beyond the roles described in this chapter, depending on the type of hospital, there can be other duties and positions available for a pharmacy technician; for example, roles dealing specifically with pediatrics, investigational drugs, and chemotherapy exist in various locations. With the advent of more specialized technology and the promotion of better patient care, more roles will develop in the future. Staying abreast of these changes and technologies is necessary to excel in these areas.

REVIEW QUESTIONS

1. What are the roles of a buyer in a health system setting?
2. What are the roles of a satellite tech in a health system setting?
3. What are the roles of a controlled substances tech in a health system setting?
4. What are the roles of a tech supervisor in a health system setting?
5. What are the roles of an automation manager in a health system setting?
6. What are the roles of a medication reconciliation tech in a health system setting?
7. List some requirements to advance into a specialty technician role in a hospital.
8. Compare the different positions in this chapter. Which one is most appealing? Least? Explain your answers.

REFERENCES

Barreto, J., Ebert, S., Maier, D., & Wooton, T. (2008, October. 23). Medication reconciliation and pharmacy technicians: Utilizing pharmacy technicians to support the medication reconciliation process. Retrieved from http://www.ashp.org/DocLibrary/MemberCenter/Webinars/Webinar20081023.aspx

O'Neal, B. (2011). Managing diversion and diverters. *Pharmacy Purchasing and Products*, 8(5), 42. Retrieved from http://www.pppmag.com/article/893/May_2011/Managing_Diversion_and_Diverters/

Siegel, J. (2010, December). In Ryan Forrey (Chair), *Code n: A multidisciplinary approach to diversion intervention*. 2010 midyear clinical meeting, Anaheim, CA. Retrieved from Amphetamines, Barbiturates, and Cocaine: The ABCs of Drug Diversion Detection and Prevention.

CHAPTER 9

Medication Safety

LEARNING OBJECTIVES

Upon completion of this chapter, you will be able to

1. Describe the nature of medication safety and its importance to pharmacy technicians
2. Identify different types of medication errors that can occur in the pharmacy
3. Analyze different scenarios and classify types of medication errors
4. List the different major organizations that deal with medication safety
5. Understand terms associated with medication errors
6. Identify different methods to prevent medication errors

KEY TERMS

Adverse drug event (ADE)

Adverse drug reaction (ADR)

Food and Drug Administration Adverse Event Reporting System (FAERS)

Institute for Safe Medication Practices (ISMP)

Medication error

Medication misadventure

Medmarx

MedWatch

National Coordinating Council for Medication Error Reporting and Prevention (NCC MERP)

Sentinel event

Standardized order set

Tall man letters

The Joint Commission (TJC)

INTRODUCTION

Pharmacy technicians play a very important role in medication safety. There are numerous areas in a hospital where medication errors can occur, not just the pharmacy department. To help reduce the occurrence of these errors, it is necessary to learn the different aspects that can affect dispensing accuracy. Terminology dealing with medication errors is also explained. Various methods of preventing and reporting errors are also discussed.

ORGANIZATIONS

There are several major organizations involved with the prevention of medication errors in the United States. The goal of these groups is to try and reduce the number of medication errors that occur in all healthcare settings. Many of the procedures, operations, and technology that exist in a hospital pharmacy today were created or guided by suggestions and recommendations from these organizations.

Institute for Safe Medication Practices

The **Institute for Safe Medication Practices (ISMP)** was created in 1975 and is the only organization of its kind that is a nonprofit entity. According to its website, its primary goal is to use its extensive experience "in helping healthcare practitioners keep patients safe, and [it] continues to lead efforts to improve the medication use process. The organization is known and respected worldwide as the premier resource for impartial, timely, and accurate medication safety information" (Institute for Safe Medication Practices, 2012).

ISMP is continuously expanding its knowledge of medication errors and offers strategies to correct or improve how pharmacies dispense medications. It publishes a newsletter that highlights the newest challenges to medication safety. It also has a national reporting system for medication errors. ISMP has a wealth of printed materials available that list the most common errors and strategies for dealing with them. The institute has many online resources available as well, including continuing education activities and other tools and resources. Live workshops and conferences are also offered.

The National Coordinating Council for Medication Error Reporting and Prevention

The **National Coordinating Council for Medication Error Reporting and Prevention (NCC MERP)** was created at the request of the U.S. Pharmacopeia

(USP) in 1995. The USP sets standards for the identity, strength, quality, and purity of medicines in the United States.

What is interesting about NCC MERP is that it is not a single organization, but a group of many other national organizations. These groups are very diverse, covering practically every aspect of health care. The group currently has 27 member organizations, including such recognized bodies as The Joint Commission, the American Society of Health-System Pharmacists, and the American Medical Association.

NCC MERP offers recommendations on error reduction, and policies on how to handle errors when they do occur. These recommendations and policies cover a wide range of healthcare settings and types. Because so many organizations contribute to NCC MERP, its analyses and recommendations are very comprehensive, taking into account the big picture and how one change or policy can affect many other departments or processes.

The Joint Commission

This organization was formerly known as the Joint Commission on the Accreditation of Healthcare Organizations (JCAHO). Its name has now been changed to simply **The Joint Commission (TJC)**. This nonprofit organization evaluates hospitals to determine whether they are complying with federal safety regulations and meeting certain minimum standards of patient care. On the organization's website, its mission statement is "to continuously improve health care for the public, in collaboration with other stakeholders, by evaluating health care organizations and inspiring them to excel in providing safe and effective care of the highest quality and value" (The Joint Commission, 2012).

Although not its only goal, medication safety is a large priority for the commission. TJC regularly visits hospitals and surveys their processes to ensure compliance. Many of the processes and policies looked at during these visits include medication preparation, dispensing, and administration. NCC MERP and ISMP offer *suggestions* on ways to improve medication safety. The Joint Commission is slightly different in that it can enforce compliance by control of accreditation. Its minimum standards of care must be met to maintain a hospital's accreditation. For this reason alone, many of the changes in procedures or methods of medication handling often are implemented because of a new standard from TJC. The pharmacy department does not want to give surveyors a reason to withdraw or not grant accreditation to the hospital. So if a new policy is instated, it may be because of a new Joint Commission standard of care.

DEFINITIONS

To understand how errors occur, as well as the means to prevent them, you must understand some of the terminology associated with medication safety and how they are related. Similar to classifications for medications, these terms can describe errors broadly and also be very specific, depending on what is being discussed.

A **medication error** is defined by NCC MERP (2012) as "any preventable event that may cause or lead to inappropriate medication use or patient harm while the medication is in the control of the healthcare professional, patient, or consumer." Many factors and aspects of the hospital pharmacy distribution system can lead to a medication error.

An **adverse drug reaction (ADR)** is a response to a drug that is noxious and unintended and that occurs at normal doses for said drug. This can be confused with the definition of a side effect; however, side effects are responses to drugs that are already known to occur and are documented. ADRs tend to be reactions that are not listed in the side effect profile for a given medication. If a patient was given diphenhydramine, for instance, and suddenly became violently nauseous, it would be considered an ADR, because nausea is not on the side effect listing for this drug and was unanticipated.

An **adverse drug event (ADE)** is any injury resulting from the use of a drug. This can include ADRs, but also overdoses and dose reductions or discontinuations. If a drug was discontinued and the patient had a bad reaction as a result, this could be considered an ADE.

An interesting umbrella term used by pharmacy to cover all of these hazards, both known and unknown, is **medication misadventure**. This term is used often by pharmacy professionals when describing medication errors and methods to reduce or prevent them.

IMPORTANCE AND RELEVANCE

Medication errors are in the public spotlight more than ever before, with the media highlighting several severe and dramatic instances of deadly or life-threatening cases that have occurred. Even though these types of occurrences may be in the minority of overall medications dispensed, due to the increased attention of the public sector this topic is high on the agenda for most institutions.

In particular, the number and types of errors that are taking place can be and, in most cases have been, prevented by the pharmacy technician. Many errors have also been attributed to technician mistakes. The most common reasoning provided to the industry and the public at large is that they did not receive enough training. This is why there has been such a drive toward formalized education for all technicians and completion of national certification testing. Many hospitals currently only hire nationally certified technicians, or have specific job titles for those who have the certified pharmacy technician (CPhT) designation.

By making fewer mistakes and catching medication errors before they occur, a pharmacy technician will be well respected by their peers and supervisors. They will also improve their perspective on the impact that we have in the dispensing process.

ERROR CATEGORIES

Medication errors can be broken down into several categories by type. It is important to note that an error often may be a combination of several types. These are not the only types or categories that exist, but the most common. By understanding the different categories of error that can occur, a pharmacy technician is more aware of how they can make a mistake. They will also increase the chance of catching a mistake made by others. This greater awareness makes the technician more valuable to the pharmacist and pharmacy department.

The American Society of Health-System Pharmacists published a document titled "Guidelines on Preventing Medication Errors in Hospitals" (American Society of Health-System Pharmacists, 1993) that provides many useful strategies for all employees in the facility. Its definitions of the different types of medication errors can be seen in **Table 9-1**. The following sections discuss these in more detail and provide some basic methods to prevent them.

Prescribing Error

Many hospitals have pharmacy technicians input medication orders into the computer system for pharmacist verification. If their translation of the order into the system isn't accurate, the pharmacist may not catch the discrepancy before verification. As shown in Table 9-1, if the prescriber's handwriting is not legible, it is not the fault of the pharmacy technician. It *is* their responsibility to get clarification, however. When dealing with medication orders, the best general principle is "when in doubt, check it out." Making an assumption is the absolute worst thing a technician can do when entering a difficult-to-read order.

Table 9-1 Types of Medication Errors[a]

Type	Definition
Prescribing error	Incorrect drug selection (based on indications, contraindications, known allergies, existing drug therapy, and other factors), dose, dosage form, quantity, route, concentration, rate of administration, or instructions for use of a drug product ordered or authorized by physician (or other legitimate prescriber); illegible prescriptions or medication orders that lead to errors that reach the patient
Omission error[b]	The failure to administer an ordered dose to a patient before the next scheduled dose, if any
Wrong time error	Administration of medication outside a predefined time interval from its scheduled administration time (this interval should be established by each individual healthcare facility)
Unauthorized drug error[c]	Administration to the patient of medication not authorized by a legitimate prescriber for the patient
Improper dose error[d]	Administration to the patient of a dose that is greater than or less than the amount ordered by the prescriber or administration of duplicate doses to the patient (i.e., one or more dosage units in addition to those that were ordered)
Wrong dosage-form error[e]	Administration to the patient of a drug product in a different dosage form than ordered by the prescriber
Wrong drug-preparation error[f]	Drug product incorrectly formulated or manipulated before administration
Wrong administration-technique error[g]	Inappropriate procedure or improper technique in the administration of a drug
Deteriorated drug error[h]	Administration of a drug that has expired or for which the physical or chemical dosage-form integrity has been compromised
Monitoring error	Failure to review a prescribed regimen for appropriateness and detection of problems, or failure to use appropriate clinical or laboratory data for adequate assessment of patient response to prescribed therapy

Table 9-1 (*Continued*)

Type	Definition
Compliance error	Inappropriate patient behavior regarding adherence to a prescribed medication regimen
Other medication error	Any medication error that does not fall into one of the above predefined categories

Source: Reproduced from American Society of Hospital Pharmacists, "ASHP guidelines on preventing medication errors in hospitals," Am J Hosp Pharm. 1993; 50:305-14.

[a] The categories may not be mutually exclusive because of the multidisciplinary and multifactorial nature of medication errors.
[b] Assumes no prescribing error. Excluded would be (1) a patient's refusal to take the medication or (2) a decision not to administer the dose because of recognized contraindications. If an explanation for the omission is apparent (e.g., patient was away from nursing unit for tests or medication was not available), that reason should be documented in the appropriate records.
[c] This would include, for example, a wrong drug, a dose given to the wrong patient, unordered drugs, and doses given outside a stated set of clinical guidelines or protocols.
[d] Excluded would be (1) allowable deviations based on preset ranges established by individual healthcare organizations in consideration of measuring devices routinely provided to those who administer drugs to patients (e.g., not administering a dose based on a patient's measured temperature or blood glucose level) or other factors such as conversion of doses expressed in the apothecary system to the metric system and (2) topical dosage forms for which medication orders are not expressed quantitatively.
[e] Excluded would be accepted protocols (established by the pharmacy and therapeutics committee or its equivalent) that authorize pharmacists to dispense alternate dosage forms for patients with special needs (e.g., liquid formulations for patients with nasogastric tubes or those who have difficulty swallowing), as allowed by state regulations.
[f] This would include, for example, incorrect dilution or reconstitution, mixing drugs that are physically or chemically incompatible, and inadequate product packaging.
[g] This would include doses administered (1) via the wrong route (different from the route prescribed), (2) via the correct route but at the wrong site (e.g., left eye instead of right), and (3) at the wrong rate of administration.
[h] This would include, for example, administration of expired drugs and improperly stored drugs.

Omission Error

This particular error usually falls under the nursing department. A pharmacy technician can also be responsible in whole or in part, depending on the circumstances involved. For example, let's say a medication was out of stock in the dispensing cabinet, or missing from the medication cart. If pharmacy was notified of the missing med, and a technician did not correct the problem in a timely fashion, it could lead to an omission error. Understand that promptness should be the norm when addressing missing medication requests, not the exception.

Wrong Time Error

This can also fall under the domain of pharmacy if medication is not dispensed in the time frame it should be. It can also occur from lack of follow-through with requests. If a call is received by a pharmacy technician but then forgotten due to a hectic workday, the medication may not be given within its specified dosing schedule.

Unauthorized Drug Error

There are many ways in which a pharmacy technician can either cause or prevent this type of error. If an incorrect drug is loaded into a dispensing cabinet or a medication cart, a nurse may not catch it before administering it to the patient. If a medication order is received by the pharmacy and inadvertently entered into the wrong patient's profile, it would look legitimate to the nurse, but in reality be an unauthorized drug error. A pharmacy technician can be mindful of drugs that look out of place on a patient profile, or look different than all of the other drugs loaded in a given pocket of a dispensing cabinet.

Improper Dose Error

The most common way a pharmacy technician can facilitate an improper dose error is when compounding IV solutions. Miscalculations during preparation can severely over- or underdose a patient. Poor technique when physically preparing the medication can deliver the wrong amount into the IV bag, even if the calculations are correct. Double- or even triple-checking calculations and practicing good aseptic manipulations minimize the chances of this type of error.

Wrong Dosage-Form Error

When entering medication orders into the pharmacy patient profile, it is typical to view all of the available formulations of a medication on the computer screen, and then select the proper one to complete the order (see **Figure 9-1**). It is very easy to accidentally select the wrong version of the medication intended. This could happen by a mere twitch of the hand when clicking on the mouse button during drug selection. This slip could be the difference between selecting aspirin tablets and instead choosing an aspirin suppository. Which would the patient most likely have preferred? Technicians should be cognizant of the ease in which a selection error can occur.

It is more difficult to make a selection mistake when pulling medications off of the shelf in the pharmacy department, at least in most cases. There are opportunities for error here as well, however. An example would be an antibiotic topical. Creams and ointments are different dose forms. Suspensions vary from solutions. In many cases a drug will exist in the same strength in multiple dose forms (**Figure 9-2**). Be aware when filling to check the dose form for these almost identical drug formulations.

Medication Lookup

Drug	Dose Form	Strength
SYNTHROID 125 MCG TABLET	TABLET	125MCG
SYNTHROID 150 MCG TABLET	TABLET	150MCG
SYNTHROID 175 MCG TABLET	TABLET	175MCG
SYNTHROID 200 MCG TABLET	TABLET	200MCG
SYNTHROID 200 MCG VIAL	VIAL	200MCG
SYNTHROID 25 MCG TABLET	TABLET	25MCG
SYNTHROID 300 MCG TABLET	TABLET	300MCG
SYNTHROID 50 MCG TABLET	TABLET	50MCG
SYNTHROID 500 MCG VIAL	VIAL	500MCG
SYNTHROID 75 MCG TABLET	TABLET	75MCG
SYNTHROID 88 MCG TABLET	TABLET	88MCG

FIGURE 9-1 Medication selection screen options.

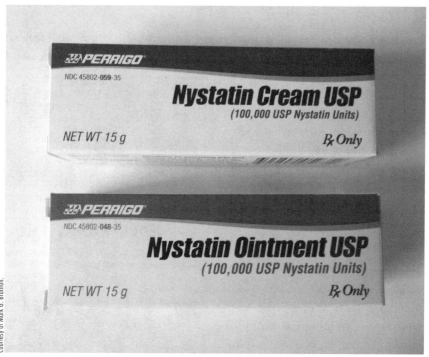

Courtesy of Mark G. Brunton.

FIGURE 9-2 An example of the same drug strength in different dose forms.

Wrong Drug-Preparation Error

Pharmacy technicians who practice poor aseptic technique or do not follow instructions carefully can cause this type of error. If a pathogen is introduced into an IV preparation during compounding, this is how the error would be classified. Another example would be reconstitution of a medication with the wrong type or amount of diluent. As with the other errors listed, never *assume* the correct method of preparation for a medication. If the correct method is not already known, seek clarification.

Wrong Administration-Technique Error

The administration of medications to patients is the responsibility of nurses. As part of the healthcare team, a pharmacy technician can have an impact on this type of error. For example, an IV drug named Mannitol has a filter that must be used when administering to a patient. It is often the responsibility of the pharmacy to provide the filter when delivering the medication to the nursing unit. If a technician was to forget to include the filter, and a nurse was not familiar with the need for that particular drug, this could lead to a wrong administration-technique error.

Deteriorated Drug Error

If a drug is not stored in its required temperature range, the medication may no longer be effective or may lose potency (**Figure 9-3**). Many drugs cannot be stored where they can be exposed to light (**Figure 9-4**). Certain drugs can break down into toxic components when they are expired. Expiration date review and refrigerator temperature verification are generally not the highest priorities in a busy workday. In order to avoid this type of error, however, they must be done.

Monitoring Error

This type of error generally is prevented by pharmacist clinical reviews and warning screens during order-entry procedures. One area in which a pharmacy technician may be involved with monitoring is the emerging medication reconciliation role. By accurately

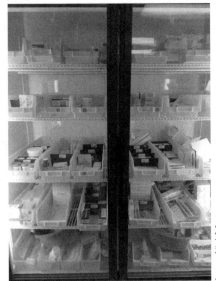

FIGURE 9-3 Refrigerated medications.

Courtesy of Mark G. Brunton.

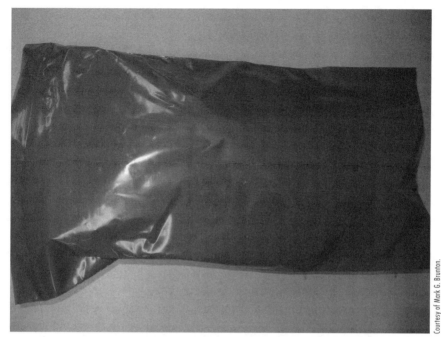

Courtesy of Mark G. Brunton.

FIGURE 9-4 An amber-colored bag can protect a light-sensitive medication from deterioration.

reviewing and determining a patient's medication regimen upon admission, a pharmacy technician can identify and prevent not only a monitoring error, but also many of the other listed errors.

Compliance Error

This type of error is much more common in a community pharmacy setting because the patient has control over the administration of his own medications. This type of error can occur in a hospital setting if a patient refuses to take his medication when it is administered by a nurse. The role of pharmacists in some hospitals can include counseling patients on proper medication use before they are discharged. If this was done incorrectly, or a patient misunderstood the instructions, then it could also lead to a compliance error.

Other Medication Error

While the above listed error categories cover many areas, they are not the only types of errors that can occur. Hospitals across the country can have many differences in the policies, procedures, and technology that they employ. These differences in their many combinations can lead to an error that does not fall into any of the categories above, and therefore would be classified as "other." A pharmacy technician with good awareness of medication safety principles can work to anticipate other types of errors that could occur, and take steps to prevent them. Being vigilant and focused can help to prevent all types of medication errors.

ERROR CAUSES

There are several major categories of causes for medication errors. Although not true for every occurrence, the majority of the medication error types that have been discussed can be linked to one or more of the following causes:

- *Technical failures:* These occur when the technology used to facilitate pharmacy operations does not operate as intended. This could be due to a mechanical malfunction or improper use by an employee. Proper maintenance of equipment and adequate training of personnel are counters to this type of failure.
- *Human failures:* These failures are at the individual level, and require personal accountability. If a technician assumes they know what a prescription says without verification, or does not check an expiration date before dispensing, they are guilty of a human failure. Holding oneself accountable for errors, and being prepared and well-rested all contribute to preventing this type of failure. See the "Tips and Tricks" section of this chapter for more on this subject.
- *Organizational failures:* Failures in the policies and procedures of a facility can cause many different types of medication errors to occur. The very structure of a department's operations, or lack of one, can contribute to decreased medication safety. Identifying weaknesses in the steps of a process or workflow is the first step in dealing with this type of failure. The next step would be to suggest an alternative. Some of the best pharmacy technicians have implemented outstanding processes and solutions by simply starting off with, "What if we tried it this way?"

A technician with good critical thinking skills can look at an error that has occurred, identify the causes, and suggest a method to prevent it from happening again.

TIPS AND TRICKS
Eyes Only

Many times the reality of the scope of medication errors is shocking to a student or new technician. This can lead to discouragement or fear about being in the field and making a potentially life-threatening mistake. Fear is not bad, if it is used in the right way. Debilitating fear is practically useless. A healthy fear is one that keeps you on your toes, but does not cause you to freeze up. This optimizes your focus and allows for safer medication dispensing and preparation.

To master your fears, the first thing to understand is that everyone makes mistakes. It is expected. The key is to learn from the mistake and not make the same one twice. A good philosophy and mindset to utilize is the "eyes only" perception. This strategy is to always assume that yours are the only eyes that will be looking at a given preparation or dispensed drug. Acting like there is no pharmacist verification will facilitate thorough review of the preparation before, during, and after it is completed. Assuming that your eyes are the only ones checking an order ensures that you are doing everything possible to make sure it is correct, because there is no safety net. Of course there is, but the key is not to rely on it.

METHODS OF PREVENTION

Now that you understand some of the different types of errors and causes of them, we can examine different strategies and tactics to help decrease them. Many of the following principles and policies are in use every day in most hospitals across the country. Methods of prevention can be classified into two general categories, personal and facility based.

Facility-Based Methods

The mechanisms and practices of a hospital pharmacy that are universal to all of the department's employees can be classified as facility-based methods of prevention. Whether uniquely created within a particular facility or implemented because of recommendations from outside organizations, these practices are very common.

Tall Man Lettering

The Food and Drug Administration (FDA), ISMP, and TJC all recommend the use of tall man lettering in hospital pharmacies. Many generic drug names are very similar in their spelling. They may have the same starting and ending letters, and roughly the same amount of letters total. When looked at casually or in a hurried fashion, these similar names are very often confused with each other. **Tall man letters** are letters within these names that are printed in capitals in order to highlight differences to the reader. Whenever someone uses ALL CAPS in a written message or text, it conveys the impression of SHOUTING. In the same fashion, tall man letters "shout out" the differences in similar drug names. This format is seen on labeling for bins on pharmacy shelves and many other storage locations in the facility. **Table 9-2** shows some examples of tall man letters for some drugs, as listed by ISMP. A more comprehensive list is available on the ISMP website (www.ismp.org).

Standardized Order Sets

In various departments in the hospital, there are many drug therapy regimens that follow very common dosing patterns. Rather than have the doctor write out

Table 9-2 FDA-Approved List of Generic Drug Names with Tall Man Letters

Drug Name with Tall Man Letters	Often Confused With
acetaZOLAMIDE	acetoHEXAMIDE
buPROPion	busPIRone
chlorproMAZINE	chlorproPAMIDE
clomiPHENE	clomiPRAMINE
cycloSERINE	cycloSPORINE
DAUNOrubicin	DOXOrubicin
dimenhyDRINATE	diphenhydrAMINE
DOBUTamine	DOPamine

Source: Data from Institute for Safe Medication Practices, "ISMP updates its list of drug name pairs with TALL man letters," ISMP Medication Safety Alert! November 18, 2011.

the same orders for every patient admitted or every time a common procedure is performed, standardized orders can be used. A **standardized order set** is a printed set of orders for procedures or medications commonly done in a given setting (see **Figure 9-5**). The doctor selects from the available printed options. This is equivalent to ordering from a menu at a restaurant, rather than writing your own food order for the waitress. There is much less room for confusion or misinterpretation when ordering from the menu. These order sets can be either printed or in an electronic format.

Personal-Based Methods

Human beings are prone to make mistakes for different reasons. At the most basic level, we require sufficient sleep in order to function at a high level of alertness. Not resting well can lead to more errors at work, and is something to avoid if at all possible in pharmacy technician practice. General health should be maintained with proper diet and exercise. Outside stressors should be minimized while on the job to allow for proper focus and attention to medication dispensing duties.

Culture of Safety

An organization's culture is defined as its shared attitudes, values, goals, and practices. Hospitals are constantly striving for a culture of safety for the patient. This includes medication safety. It would not be the responsibility of the pharmacy technician to create this culture . . . or would it? All it takes is one person to set an example that others can follow. That person can be anyone in a facility—a doctor, nurse, or pharmacy technician. It is always better to set a higher standard rather than follow a lower one.

One of the most common elements of a medication error is assumption. There are usually so many safeguards and sets of eyes looking at a particular medication that errors have almost zero chance of being administered to the patient. Note the use of the word *almost*. It is not uncommon for a nurse, even subconsciously, to assume that pharmacy did not make an error, because 9 times out of 10 they don't. It is not uncommon for the pharmacy, even subconsciously, to assume that *if* a mistake happened, a nurse would surely spot it and correct it. This is exactly when an error will occur.

In a facility with a strong culture of safety, every staff member is encouraged to speak up if they see an area that may impact patient care or lead to an error. This could be a faulty process or another opportunity for a mistake to be made. A pharmacy technician can foster this culture by setting an example, rather than

Hospital
"Code Stroke" Order Set

| Please place within box |
| Patient Label |

Check box to activate order if applicable		
Date and time	Admission information	If patient presents with new neurological deficits call "Code Stroke" overhead. Estimate time of symptoms onset (time last seen normal): _____ Time patient presented to ER: _____ Medication allergies: _____ Weight: _____kg (estimated)
Date and time	Notifications	Notify Nursing Supervisor at _____ Notify Radiology/CT technician (if not in house)—paged/called at _____ Notify Laboratory staff (if not in house)—paged/called at _____
Date and time	Interventions/ treatments	Take immediately from triage to bed. VS and neuro checks every 15 minutes (Use Cincinnatti Stroke Scale and Glascow Coma Scale). Continuous ECG monitoring. Continuous pulse oximetry. Oxygen @ 2L by nasal cannula to keep O_2 sat $\geq$ 92% Place 2 peripheral IV's and saline lock—at least one 18G. Obtain a bedside glucose measurement.
Date and time	Prevention of aspiration	NPO Keep head of bed elevated to 30–45 degrees at all times. Complete a Nurse Swallow Evaluation (don't delay thrombolytics to do this).
Date and time	Labs	CBC BMP PT/INR, PTT Other: _____
Date and time	Diagnostic tests	STAT non-contrast CT brain scan—Reason: Acute CNS event—"Code Stroke" [Goal: <25 min from ER arrival to CT] [Goal: <45 min to CT results] 12-lead ECG STAT (don't delay CT) CXR portable STAT (don't delay CT) Other: _____
Date and time	Blood pressure medications	Ischemic Stroke BP Management: If SBP > 185 or DBP > 110 Target SBP is $\geq$ 120 and $\leq$ 180 and DBP is $\geq$ 60 and $\leq$ 105 ❏ Labetalol 10 mg IV; May repeat every 10 minutes × 3 doses. If unresponsive to Labetalol or other contraindications to beta blocker effect (asthma or bradycardia) give: ❏ (0.2mg/ml) by continuous IV infusion. Start at 5mg/hour. May increase 2.5mg/hour every 5–15 minutes, maximum 15 mg/hour.

Physician Signature: _____

RN Signature: _____

FIGURE 9-5 Example of a standardized order set.

**Hospital
"Code Stroke" Order Set**

		Please place within box Patient Label

Date and time	PRN medications	❑ Acetaminophen 650mg PR every 4 hours PRN Temp ≥ 99.6 F (37.5C) or mild pain ≤ 3 Or if NPO or otherwise cannot tolerate po meds, then: ❑ Acetaminophen (OFIRMEV) _____mg IV every 6 hours PRN temp ≥ 99.6°F (recommended dose: • >13 years and > 50 kg = 1,000mg every 6 hours, • < 50kg = 15mg/kg every 6 hours—max daily dose = 4gm/24 hours) ❑ Ondansetron (Zofran) 4mg IV every 6 hours PRN nausea or vomiting
Date and time	Peptic ulcer prophylaxis	Protonix 40mg IV daily Other: _____

Date and time	t-PA decision	Complete t-PA Inclusion/Exclusion Criteria Form (if not already done)
		t-PA candidate = Ischemic Stroke within 4.5 hours of symptom onset and without contraindications.
		    (Goal: <60 minutes from ER arrival to t-PA)
		Decision:
		❑ Will not be administered due to symptoms delays > 4.5 hours
		❑ Will be administered with the following dosing:
		    t-PA (Alteplase) dosing: 0.9mg/kg = _____mg total dose (max dose = 90mg)
		    • Administer 10% of total dose as IV bolus over 1 minute (_____mg) and then 90% of total dose (_____mg) as IV infusion over 1 hour.
		    • Report any changes in vital signs, neurological status, or any bleeding to physician immediately.
		Intracranial Hemorrhage Management Guidelines During and After t-PA Infusion
		If clinical suspicion of ICH present, notify physician immediately.
		Order: _____

Date and time	Intracranial hemorrhage	• CT Head STAT—Reason: R/O CNS bleed S/P tPA • CBC, PT, INR, PTT, Fibrinogen STAT • T&C 4 units PRBCs, 4 units cryoprecipitated fibrinogen, 2 Units FFP (Use Blood Transfusion Order Sheet) If CT Head shows hemorrhage and clinical situation justifies, then: • If fibrinogen < 50, administer 5 units cryoprecipitated fibrinogen • If PT > 24sec or PTT > 50sec, and fibrinogen > 80mg, then administer 2 units FFP • If platelets < 50,000, administer 1 unit platelet pheresis pack If any blood product administered, order PT, PTT. Contact stroke neurologist to evaluate for transfer.
Date and time	Other	_____ _____ _____ _____

Physician Signature: _____

RN Signature: _____

FIGURE 9-5 (*Continued*)

following one. By always being attentive and aware of medication safety, a pharmacy technician can be the one to catch errors rather than cause them.

Reporting

It is said that we should learn from our mistakes. Never is this truer than in the case of medication safety. Moreover, it is a best practice to share our mistakes with the rest of the field so other healthcare workers and institutions can learn from them as well. There are many databases that collect information on the nature of medication errors that occur. These can be systems based within the facility, and also at the state and national level.

One of the largest fears of healthcare workers is that of being punished for making a mistake. That is why most of these systems have the option of reporting anonymously. It is not *who* made the error that is important, but *how* and *why* it occurred in order to create strategies to prevent it from happening again. A pharmacy technician should never be afraid to admit making a mistake, and should do so in order to help prevent others from making the same one.

An example of an institution-specific reporting system is **Medmarx**, a program a hospital can purchase to document electronically when errors occur (Medmarx International Reporting, 2012). Computers across the facility have the program loaded, and any employee can use it to report errors. This information can be used to improve safety within the hospital, and the data collected are specific to that institution. Medmarx also collects these data from all of its accounts, and formulates strategies and suggestions based on the results for dissemination.

The Food and Drug Administration has a national reporting system known as the **FDA Adverse Event Reporting System (FAERS)** that is used to determine issues that may be corrected by the manufacturer. Concerns such as labeling deficiencies, counterfeit products, or drugs of poor quality can be corrected using this system. The FDA also runs the **MedWatch** program, which consists of newsletters and video broadcasts that can be viewed from its website (U.S. Food and Drug Administration, 2012). The goal of MedWatch is to inform both healthcare practitioners and the general public about safety concerns regarding medications. It is very useful for keeping abreast of the most current types of errors and safety concerns that develop in the field.

The Joint Commission has a very specific reporting system and protocol for hospitals, and it is highly useful for increasing medication safety. When errors occur, or almost occur, the result is not always life threatening to the patient. If a dose of Motrin is missed, for example, it is unlikely that the patient will suffer instant cardiac arrest. Unfortunately, there *are* errors that are very deadly or dangerous and do happen in the hospital setting. The Joint Commission calls these types of errors **sentinel events**. According to TJC's definition, a sentinel event is "an unexpected occurrence involving death or serious physical or psychological injury, or the risk thereof" (The Joint Commission, 2012). The term *sentinel* means literally to keep watch. This protocol ensures that when a life-threatening or very dangerous event happens, the hospital will take measures to correct it.

The Joint Commission's sentinel event protocol states that if an event occurs, the hospital must investigate the root cause of the error, and develop an action plan that will prevent it from happening again. The hospital is encouraged to report the incident to TJC as soon as possible so it can be input into its national sentinel events database, but this is not required. However, if a sentinel event occurs and is not handled appropriately by the hospital, it may affect future accreditation status by The Joint Commission.

SUMMARY

Medication errors are a challenge for every hospital. Every employee has the responsibility and opportunity to prevent them from occurring. New technologies and processes are being developed all the time in order to reduce error rates even further. No system is 100% perfect, however. A good pharmacy technician is aware of the nature of medication errors, and strives to do the best they can to perform their duties with as much diligence and precision as they can, every day.

REVIEW QUESTIONS

1. Name two organizations involved in the reduction of medication errors. How do they go about this goal?
2. What is the definition of a medication error?
3. List four types of medication errors, and provide examples of each. Are these able to be caused by a technician in health system practice?
4. Give an example of how a medication error can involve more than one category.
5. A patient had an order written for $MgSO_4$, and was administered morphine sulfate. Which type of error is this?
6. If a patient acquires an infection after receiving a poorly made IV preparation, which type of error is this?

7. Give an example of a human failure error as a technician.
8. Give an example of a technical failure in the pharmacy department that can lead to a medication error.
9. List three methods for reducing medication errors
10. Name three personal practices that can be used to reduce the chances of making a medication error.

REFERENCES

American Society of Health-System Pharmacists. (1993). ASHP guidelines on preventing medication errors in hospitals. Retrieved from http://www.ashp.org/s_ashp/docs/files/MedMis_Gdl_Hosp.pdf

Institute for Safe Medication Practices. (2012). FDA and ISMP lists of look-alike drug names with recommended tall man letters. Retrieved from http://www.ismp.org/Tools/tallmanletters.pdf

The Joint Commission. (2012). Retrieved from http://www.jointcommission.org

Medmarx International Reporting. (2012). Retrieved from https://www.medmarx.com

National Coordinating Council for Medication Error Prevention. (2012). Retrieved from http://www.nccmerp.org

U.S. Food and Drug Administration. (2012). Drugs. Retrieved from http://www.fda.gov/Drugs/default.htm

PART 4

Informatics and Technology

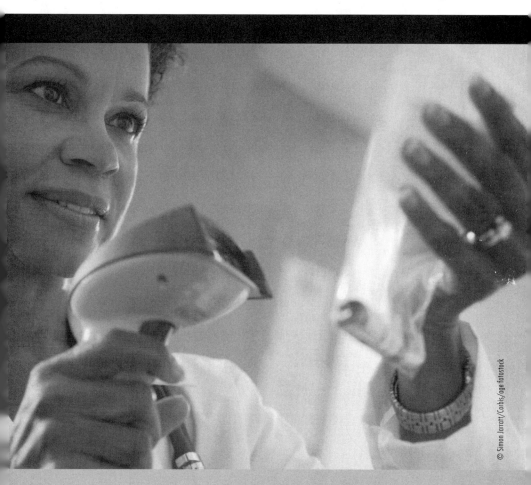

© Simon Jarratt/Corbis/age fotostock

CHAPTER 10

Health System Software and Equipment

LEARNING OBJECTIVES

Upon completion of this chapter, you will be able to

1. Describe the function of health system software applications
2. Identify common peripheral devices used by other departments besides pharmacy
3. Recognize situations that occur due to software and peripheral interaction with the pharmacy department

KEY TERMS

Admissions
ADT system
Computer on wheels (COW)
Computerized physician order entry (CPOE)
Discharges
Electronic health record (EHR)

Electronic medication administration record (EMAR)
Hospital information systems (HIS)
Patient ID
Transfers

INTRODUCTION

It is absolutely essential to be able to utilize pharmacy software and equipment to complete daily job duties. A pharmacy technician should also have an introductory understanding of the different software and equipment that are used by *other* departments in the hospital. These programs and machines interact with the pharmacy department in many ways, and may require troubleshooting in some instances. By knowing what nurses, doctors, and other hospital staff use to complete their daily duties, you can help address any problems as they arise in a more efficient manner.

ADT SYSTEM

The main software used by the rest of the hospital is generally referred to as an **ADT system**. ADT is an acronym that stands for admissions, discharges, and transfers. It is similar to the patient profiling software used by the pharmacy, in that it catalogs patient information. The types of information that it deals with are much broader than pharmacy software, however. The ADT system communicates directly with the pharmacy software server, constantly transferring and updating information on patients within the facility (see **Figure 10-1**). Note the direction of information transfer. ADT information updates pharmacy software, not the other way around. A pharmacy technician cannot discharge a patient or transfer him to a new location and expect it

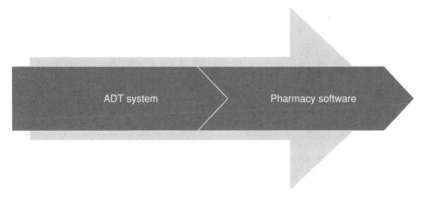

FIGURE 10-1 Information transfer between the ADT system and pharmacy.

to update the ADT database, but any of these changes made on the ADT side will automatically update the pharmacy system. Let's look at the components or aspects of the ADT system.

Admissions

The admissions department handles the input of information for every person that becomes a patient of the hospital. When referring to software applications, an **admission** is the record of that information in the ADT system. Patients may enter the hospital by coming in on their own and requesting admission or they may be brought into the emergency room (ER). When a patient is admitted, certain key pieces of information are gathered and entered into their admissions record. These items are:

- *Identifying information:* This includes contact information such as address, phone number, emergency contacts, Social Security number, and so on.
- *Patient demographics:* This is information about the patient that would be used for clinical purposes, such as height, weight, preexisting medical conditions, and medication history.
- *Insurance information:* There are many different insurance plans and companies that a patient may use. This information must be accurately documented for billing purposes.

Note that these pieces of information and more are similar to what would be collected by a pharmacy technician in the retail setting. In a hospital setting, this information is already in the system for the pharmacy department to use. If a patient does not show up in the pharmacy database, one of the possible reasons is that they have not been entered into the ADT system in order for the information to have crossed over, or there is an interruption in data transfer between the two systems.

Depending on the circumstance of the admission, some information may not be entered immediately upon arrival to the facility. For example, if a patient was admitted to the ER unconscious, their allergy information may have to be acquired and entered when they wake up, or ER personnel may still be trying to measure the patient's height and weight. A pharmacy technician may have to call a nurse and have them confirm or enter in the patient's allergy information because it was not completed during the initial admissions process.

When a patient is admitted to the facility, they are assigned a unique number for the duration of their visit. This is called the patient identification number, or simply the **patient ID**. The patient ID number can be used to look up patients in the pharmacy database, and is often a preferred method for minimizing the chance of selecting the wrong patient. Two patients named Smith, John, would have different patient IDs.

Discharges

When patients leave the care of the hospital, they are considered **discharges**. Patients who are discharged from the facility are still accessible in the computer database, but their status has changed. When this transfers into the pharmacy system, any drugs that were scheduled for that patient are discontinued.

Transfers

A **transfer** occurs when a patient is moved from one location to another within the facility. This could happen due to a change in the status of the patient's condition or availability of beds. A patient being transferred into an intensive care unit (ICU) due to a worsening infection would be an example, or putting two patients into one room to accommodate an influx of new admissions.

Depending on the efficiency of the computer systems in the facility, or the quality of the interface between systems, transfers can be a common cause for minor challenges in the pharmacy department. If the facility in question uses automated dispensing cabinet (ADC) technology, nurses may have difficulty removing medications for a patient that recently was transferred to their unit. This would occur if the transfer has not processed through the ADT system to the pharmacy, and then from there to the ADC system (**Figure 10-2**).

Electronic Health Record

A patient's entire medical history can encompass many different elements, and be scattered among various healthcare providers. For example, a patient could be sent to a radiologist's office for x-rays, then to a rehabilitation specialist for therapy, followed by a consultation with a pain management

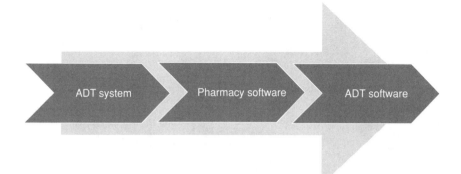

FIGURE 10-2 Delays in transfer between software systems can impede medication administration.

specialist. All of these different locations and practitioners have a portion of the patient's total treatment information. They can share this information with each other upon request, or give a copy to the patient to take with them. Admission to a hospital may not include much, or any of this data. The **electronic health record (EHR)** is a new concept and technology being implemented to streamline this process. The EHR is all of the separate components mentioned collected together and available to all healthcare providers involved at need. This is done through the communication and computing power of the Internet.

With a functioning EHR, healthcare providers are able to access a patient's complete health history while the patient is in their care. This includes information from other facilities they have been to, any blood work or lab data that have been processed, or diagnoses from specialists. This will also include allergy information and current prescribed drug history. This enables the healthcare practitioner to make a more informed and accurate decision regarding the patient's treatment, because they have access to the big picture (HealthIT.gov, n.d.b.). See **Figure 10-3** for an illustration of this concept.

The EHR is a hot topic within health care as of the time of this writing. There are many incentives for providers to implement these systems in their practice. Medicare and Medicaid will provide incentive payments to hospitals and others who use EHR technology, effectively subsidizing their cost, and also modernizing the practice of health care.

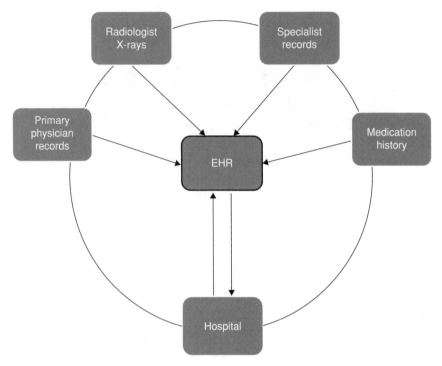

FIGURE 10-3 Information transfer relationships within the EHR.

NURSING EQUIPMENT AND SOFTWARE

Nurses also utilize the ADT system to access patient information, and there are additional equipment and programs that they use for patient care. Much of the technology currently being implemented in today's hospitals utilizes barcode devices. When a patient is admitted and given a patient ID number, this information is attached to a wristband that the patient wears the entire time they are guests of the facility (see **Figure 10-4**). On this wristband are the patient's name, ID number, and also a barcode representation of the ID.

A nurse's main responsibility is to provide a standard level of care to the patient. Administration of medications is a critical component of this goal. A nurse must document every medication given to a patient. This task was traditionally done by hand, written on a medication administration record

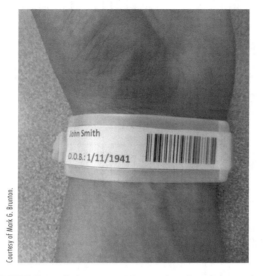

Courtesy of Mark G. Brunton.

FIGURE 10-4 A patient ID wristband with barcoding.

(see **Figure 10-5**). This record can be prone to error. The accuracy of the documentation is dependent on human accuracy and consistency, which is never 100%. If a nurse is very busy, it is not uncommon for medications to be given to the patient and not documented, or vice versa.

With the advent of bedside computing and bar coding, this potential for error can be significantly reduced. One of the pieces of equipment that is now used is commonly called a **computer on wheels (COW)** or workstation on wheels (WOW). This is a portable computer workstation that can be wheeled to each patient's bedside in order to chart and document nursing activities as they occur (see **Figure 10-6**). The COW has access to the ADT system, so the nurse can pull up a given patient's chart and notes at a moment's notice. This is useful for checking lab values, charting vital signs, and keeping detailed records of the patient's care.

A critical pharmaceutical component of the COW system is its enhancement of the medication administration process. Built into the workstation is a barcode scanner that can be used when administering medications to a patient. The process of administration is as follows:

1. A nurse scans the patient's wristband barcode to confirm identity (see **Figure 10-7**).

Medication Administration Record (MAR)

MO/YR: _____ Start/Stop Date Facility Name: _____

Medication	Start/Stop	Hour	1	2	3	4	5	6	7	8	9	10	11	12	13	14	15	16	17	18	19	20	21	22	23	24	25	26	27	28	29	30	31
	Start																																	
	Stop																																	
	Start																																	
	Stop																																	
	Start																																	
	Stop																																	
	Start																																	
	Stop																																	
	Start																																	
	Stop																																	
	Start																																	
	Stop																																	

Diet (Special instructions, e.g. texture, bite size, position, etc.):

Diagnosis:

Allergies:

Physician name:

Phone number:

Record #:

Comments:

A. Put initials in appropriate box when medication is given.
B. Circle initials when not given.
C. State reason for refusal/omission on back of form.
D. PRN Medications: Reasons given and results must be noted on back of form.
E. Legend: S = School; H = Home visit; W = Work; P = Program.

Name: _____ Date of birth: _____ Sex: _____

FIGURE 10-5 A paper Medication Administration Record (MAR).

Vital signs	1	2	3	4	5	6	7	8	9	10	11	12	13	14	15	16	17	18	19	20	21	22	23	24	25	26	27	28	29	30	31
Temperature																															
Pulse																															
Respiration																															
Weight																															

PRN and medications not administered

Date	Hour	Initials	Medication	Reason	Result

Initials	Staff Signature
1	
2	
3	
4	
5	
6	
7	
8	
9	
10	
11	
12	
13	
14	
15	
16	
17	
18	
19	

Name: MO/YR:

FIGURE 10-5 (*continued*)

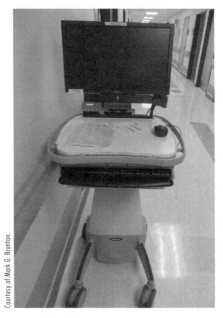

Courtesy of Mark G. Brunton.

FIGURE 10-6 Examples of Computers on Wheels (COWs) or Workstation on Wheels (WOWs).

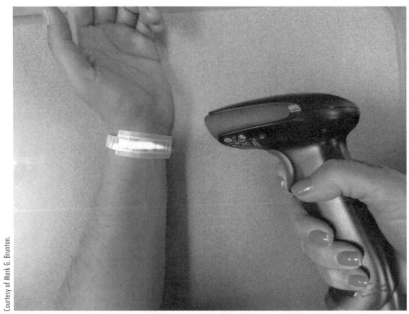

Courtesy of Mark G. Brunton.

FIGURE 10-7 Scanning a patient arm band.

2. The nurse then scans the barcode on the unit-dosed medication to confirm that the appropriate drug is being administered (see **Figure 10-8**).

3. The COW verifies the accurate medication is being given and documents the action.

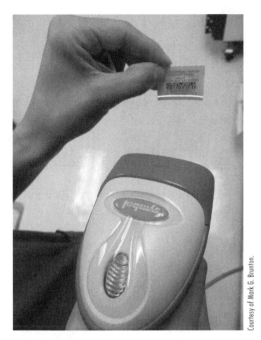

FIGURE 10-8 Scanning a medication with the COW.

If there is an error, such as having the wrong drug in hand, trying to give the drug too early, or even trying to give a drug to the wrong patient, the COW will alert the nurse of the error. This decreases the chance of a medication error significantly, because the system functions as another pair of eyes before administration.

When this process takes place, another component is also being utilized. COWs also have the ability to document the successful administration of drugs to patients as they occur, rather than having to write it out by hand later. This piece of software is referred to as an **electronic medication administration record (EMAR)**.

PHYSICIAN EQUIPMENT AND SOFTWARE

Doctors are central in determining what drives hospital operations. They are the members of the healthcare team that diagnose patient diseases and disorders, plan and order treatment and drug therapy regimens, and are ultimately accountable for the outcomes of their patients. The primary means of communication between a physician and the pharmacy in a hospital setting has always been via the medication order from a patient's chart. Pharmacists would talk to physicians on the telephone when coordinating or clarifying the specifics of a drug order for a given patient. New technologies are being developed that are having a major effect on the nature of physician/pharmacy interactions.

Computerized Physician Order Entry

There has long been a stereotype of physicians having horrible handwriting when writing prescriptions. This stereotype is also believed in the hospital setting in regards to medication orders. There is a reason for its existence, because some physicians do not have the best penmanship. Handwriting misinterpretation is a reason for many medication errors. There have been efforts to improve this area of error, going so far as to having penmanship classes in some medical schools. There is a new initiative and technology that aims to eliminate this particular source of error completely.

Computerized physician order entry (CPOE) is a new type of software program that is being implemented in hospitals across the county. Coupled with other forms of electronic information entry, this type of program allows a doctor to input their orders for a patient directly into the hospital computer system, without having to physically write an order into the patient's chart. This allows the patient's chart to be almost entirely electronic. This process has many advantages:

- *Speed:* Rather than writing an order and waiting for it to get transmitted to the appropriate department, such as pharmacy, the order is transmitted immediately to the pharmacy after the doctor enters it.
- *Accuracy:* Misinterpretation due to poor handwriting is a nonissue. The order is as clearly legible to the pharmacy as the text you are reading at this very moment. In addition, the doctor can review the patient's profile and treatment information during the order entry process, allowing for adjustments or changes to the order before it has even been completed.
- *Safety:* Much like the order entry systems used by the pharmacy department, CPOE systems have access to the patient's medical history. If there is a possibility of interaction or duplication of therapy, the physician is notified. Prior to this type of program, a pharmacist or pharmacy technician would be the first to discover these interactions and have to contact the physician for further instructions, delaying treatment for the patient. (HealthIT.gov, n.d.a.)

CPOE systems empower the physician to make better informed decisions about the course of drug therapy, and act as a second set of eyes to help prevent prescribing errors. Note that this type of system is still in its infancy, with many companies offering different versions of software to accomplish the task at hand. There are still glitches and bugs to work out, and time is needed for effective utilization of this technology. One element that is fairly standard among these programs is the menu style of order entry. The doctor does not have to enter the order into the computer from scratch; rather, there is a list of available medications to choose from, as well as standardized signa codes and additional instructions. The signa is the dosing instruction for a given medication.

Referencing Software

There is a vast amount of information regarding medications that is not necessarily known by physicians. Advances in the field of medicine far outpace the ability of any one physician to keep up with them completely. There is simply no way for a doctor to know everything about every medication on the market in terms of dosing, interaction, side effects, and so on. In the past, books such as the *Physician's Desk Reference* or *Drug Facts and Comparisons* were the main source of this knowledge for physicians. The other source would be to contact the pharmacy and ask for further information.

These sources are still in use today, but are being supplemented and in some cases replaced by the availability of alternative sources on the Internet.

Online Resources

The texts listed are still heavily used, but they are accessed more regularly from a computer. The speed with which ebooks can be loaded and searched is near instantaneous. Every computer in a nursing unit generally has Internet access, and therefore is a potential reference source. This is more advantageous than having only one or two physical copies of a text in the unit.

Online journals and other websites provide a wealth of information for doctors to draw from. These sources may also be utilized by the pharmacy department when recommending treatment or confirming medication compatibility, among other functions. Journals also have the most current information in a given field, because they publish research results and the newest available medication therapies.

Tablets and Smartphones

It has been said that yesterday's science fiction is today's science fact. It was once a fantasy to have a handheld device that could pull up any information requested for treatment of the patient. In today's realm of smartphones and iPads, this scenario is a reality, and even sitting down to an "old-fashioned" computer isn't the fastest way to look up information anymore. There are many applications that can be downloaded for tablet PCs or smartphones for use in patient care. There are even some applications actually designed to be an extension of the hospital computer system. These peripheral applications allow doctors to be out on the floor longer, rather than having to return to the nursing station to enter orders. This portability is a very exciting aspect of the technology that can be used in today's hospitals.

FULLY INTEGRATED SYSTEMS

The ADT, CPOE, and even pharmacy software programs are often collectively lumped under the term **hospital information systems (HIS)**. These different components, among others, would communicate with each other, but were separate platforms that could run independently. If there was a break in communications, it could impact or slow down the operations of the other systems. The reasons for a break in communications could be a physical malfunction, such as a server overheating or a cable being loose, but could also be a software interface problem. This would be analogous to the 13 colonies of the United States before they became a union. Although many hospitals' HIS systems still operate in this fashion, there is a growing trend towards what is known as a fully integrated model. A fully integrated hospital uses one software system for all departments. There are several different software platforms leading this initiative, with brands such as Cerner and Epic being at the forefront of this type of model.

TROUBLESHOOTING

When it comes to technology, knowing more is always better. Whether it is hardware or software, the more a pharmacy technician learns about it, the more useful they are to the department. If present during an install or implementation of a new piece of technology or software, certain actions can be very useful for a pharmacy technician.

- *Use the rep:* It is unlikely that the representative of the product being implemented will go over every possible function available. Most users of a new piece of technology will be wary of it, and it is often a challenge just to educate staff about the bare minimum in terms of function. There is no reason, however, not to go up to the rep at a convenient moment and ask, "What else can it do?" This tactic may provide information that you do not have time to implement at the outset, but knowing about it allows you to bring it up later when everyone is used to the new system.

- *Take notes:* This is one of the most overlooked and underutilized methods of retaining information in the field. No matter how much experience you may have or how smart and clever you are, there will always be some piece of information that you don't remember when learning something new. The solution is to take notes on key items or instructions that you may forget later. This also takes the burden off of your brain to remember every little detail, and allows it to be able to focus on the information being presented and actively listen.
- *Don't be afraid:* Errors, glitches, and operator mistakes are expected to happen in the first stages of an implementation process. This is the time to take the bull by the horns and try out every aspect of the new system you are working with. It is better to make a mistake and learn from it while everyone else is doing the same.
- *Go with the flow:* When new products are brought online for any department in the hospital, hiccups will occur. Start dates may be pushed back, delaying installations. Policies and procedures may change on a daily basis, adjusting for unexpected outcomes and reactions. Being able to adapt to these changes and maintain a positive attitude and mindset will make the process less traumatic for you and those around you.

SUMMARY

A whole network of devices and systems are used in a hospital setting. Nurses, doctors, and pharmacy staff all have specific programs and machines they use to deliver their aspects of patient care. There is a push towards unification of these separate systems into one single database and program for a facility.

Technology is often put on a pedestal as the means to solve all of our problems. In health care it is considered the answer to eliminating medication errors, improving patient safety, and raising the bar in terms of a patient's quality of care. This is true, to a certain extent. New technologies and innovations are always being developed that will affect operations in a hospital pharmacy.

One of my favorite statements is, "That's why we are called pharmacy *technicians*, not pharmacy I-don't-know-how-to-work-this." The technical aspect of these systems is not "What does it do?" but more "How does it work?" Understanding how hospital information services and devices interact and operate will make you a better technician, period. More importantly, understanding how to *adapt* to new systems will make you indispensable to your department and the profession at large.

REVIEW QUESTIONS

1. What is the ADT system responsible for? In what ways does it interact with pharmacy-based software?
2. In what ways does the EHR improve patient care? How would pharmacy interact with the EHR?
3. Why are COWs used in a hospital setting?
4. What is an EMAR? What is its significance to the pharmacy department?
5. Does CPOE replace the need for pharmacy staff to enter orders? Why or why not?
6. What online resources are used in pharmacy for medication information?
7. What applications are available for smartphone and tablet platforms for pharmacy?
8. How does full integration with hospital computers affect pharmacy operations?
9. Name several techniques used for effective troubleshooting.
10. What problems can occur with pharmacy and health system software that a technician might have to troubleshoot?

REFERENCES

HealthIT.gov. (n.d.a.). Core measure 1: Computerized physician order entry (CPOE) for medication orders. Retrieved from http://www.healthit.gov/providers-professionals/achieve-meaningful-use/core-measures/cpoe-meaningful-use

HealthIT.gov. (n.d.b.). Learn EHR basics. Retrieved from http://www.healthit.gov/providers-professionals/learn-ehr-basics

CHAPTER 11

Pharmacy Management Software and Peripherals

LEARNING OBJECTIVES

Upon completion of this chapter, you will be able to

1. List the primary functions of pharmacy management software
2. Understand technician operations utilizing pharmacy management software
3. Describe medication order scanning equipment and its use in a health system setting

KEY TERMS

Order set	Sig codes
Patient lookup	Turnaround time
Patient profile	Warning screens
Sig	

INTRODUCTION

A pharmacy technician in a health system setting cannot operate effectively without a computer. It is an integral part of almost every operation that may be encountered. Pharmacy software programs accomplish the printing of labels, patient lookup functions, lab data gathering, as well as many more features and capabilities.

Although many different types of programs exist, all of them have similarities in what they are designed to do. The differences lie in the methods to access these options, or are mainly superficial in nature. An example would be like using two different Internet web browsers. Both Firefox and Internet Explorer are programs that can access the Internet, and both function in similar ways, but are different programs.

The purpose of this chapter is to give an underlying structure and framework of how pharmacy software and related peripheral devices work, which will enable easier comprehension of various proprietary systems.

FUNCTIONALITY

The majority of pharmacy computer systems are based on the Windows operating system format. This means that navigation of the software utilizes standard components such as drop-down menus and pop-up windows. Scroll bars and resizing of different windows are also features of this type of interface. Navigation is done primarily using a mouse with point-and-click actions.

TECHNICIAN OPERATIONS

A pharmacy technician can perform a wide variety of activities using patient management software (**Figure 11-1**). Of those activities, several operations are performed on a daily basis. A technician can be expected to access patient profiles regularly and perform different functions therein. In many cases technicians also have responsibilities regarding order entry and clinical information gathering activities.

Patient Lookup

The first action taken by a pharmacy technician when answering telephone calls is patient lookup. **Patient lookup** is the part of the software that allows one to select a specific patient from the pharmacy software database. Several patient identifiers can be used to find a patient:

- *Last name:* By typing the last name of a patient in the search field, the software will display all patients in the facility who have that last name. Typically only the first few letters are entered before initiating a search, because that is usually enough to narrow the search results to a manageable number.

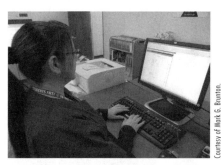

FIGURE 11-1 A technician performs many computer-related activities.

- *Patient ID number:* Each patient of the facility is issued a patient ID number upon admission. This can be used to locate a patient.
- *Unit:* It may also be possible to search for a patient by nursing unit, selecting from a list of all patients located on a certain floor, for instance.

Patient Profile

After a patient has been selected using the patient lookup function, the patient profile screen is accessed. A **patient profile** is the record of a specific patient in the facility. Many pieces of information can be accessed from the patient profile. These may include:

- *Patient demographics:* In a health system these can include age, height, weight, and allergies.
- *Medication history:* This is one of the key areas of the profile that technicians utilize in everyday practice. This section of the profile shows all of the medications that have been ordered for the patient while in the care of the facility. This includes both active or current orders, and discontinued medications.
- *Clinical data:* This information is generally related to pharmacist drug utilization review functions, such as adverse drug reactions, interactions, and contraindications. This section can also deal with lab values and test results from blood work. Some examples include hematocrit levels and creatinine clearance. Technicians are sometimes tasked with checking these values and notifying the pharmacist when certain values are within a specified range.

Charges/Credits

The charges and credits function involves billing activities for patients in the facility. The actual receiving of payment for a patient's hospital stay is handled by

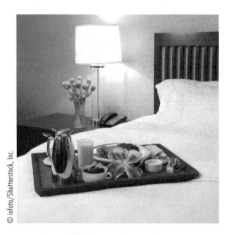

© iofoto/Shutterstock, Inc.

FIGURE 11-2 A technician improperly charging a patient would be like paying for room service a guest did not actually receive.

the hospital's billing department. This includes the cost of any medications used. This is different than a retail pharmacy setting, where technicians deal with insurance directly for payment, or deal with prescription benefits managers. This does not mean that we have no responsibility for billing in a health system setting, however. The pharmacy management software has the ability to charge patients and also issue credits for medications. These charges or credits are sent to the hospital billing department electronically to be processed. A good analogy would be like room service in a hotel (**Figure 11-2**). Room service would charge the guest for whatever food or drink was ordered, and those charges would show up on the bill at the end of the stay at the front desk.

A technician's role for charges would be to access the patient profile and charge for a specific item and quantity used. An example would be entering in crash cart charges or anesthesia tray charges. Credits are entered for a patient when a medication that was previously charged was not administered. This could be for a variety of reasons, such as if the patient was discharged, died, or the medication was discontinued. In any event, if the medication was not actually administered to the patient and has been returned to the pharmacy, it must be credited to their account so they are not charged for it.

IN THE FIELD
Charges and Credits and Bears, Oh My!

The task of charging and crediting medications can often fall on the back burner in terms of priorities in a technician's workflow. When compared to other tasks, such as preparing new orders or stat medications, delivering rounds, and answering telephones, crediting a medication that was not used is a very easy task to forget. Time should be made for it at some point in the day, however. The reality of the situation is that if medications that were not used are charged to a patient's account, it is technically fraudulent. Imagine if you stayed at a hotel on vacation, and were charged an extra $300 for a spa package that you did not actually use. Charging for medication that was not used would be the same concept.

Label Generation

This action can happen automatically when new orders are entered and verified, usually when dealing with an IV or medication not loaded in an automated dispensing cabinet (ADC). It can also be manually initiated by a technician when necessary. For example, let's say an ADC ran out of stock for a needed medication, and the nurse needed the dose stat. A technician could generate a label for a single dose, which would also generate a charge. The technician could then proceed to fill the label and, after verification, deliver it to the nurse.

Order Entry

Commonly referred to as technician order entry, this practice exists in many, but not all, hospital pharmacies. Similar to retail operations, this function is used when a technician enters medication orders into the management software. This is done to allow the pharmacist more time to perform clinical duties such as medication therapy management. Note that typically with this process, any order entered by the pharmacy technician is not active until it has undergone pharmacist review and approval. There are several elements of order entry as it pertains to pharmacy software that must be understood in order to grasp the procedure. Remember that not all software programs are the same, and these concepts may be in a different order or combined in various ways from system to system. When a medication order is received, the first step is to access the correct patient profile. Then the process of order entry can begin.

Medication Selection

Once the medication order has been deciphered, it must be entered into the profile. Medication selection is the first step in this process. The process is similar to a patient lookup. The technician would enter the first few letters of the medication to be selected. A screen would then appear with all of the available medications that fit the search criteria. There are very often multiple options of the same drug to select from; for example, there may be eight versions of Pepcid for selection. Each version could be a different strength, dose form, or unit of measure. This part of the order entry process is known to be a source of mistakes for order entry operations. Proper medication selection is imperative. Sometimes the correct option is intended for selection, but a mere twitch of the hand on the mouse could accidentally select the option directly above or below the desired field.

Sig Codes

Sig, short for *signa*, is the Latin term used in prescription writing when referring to directions for the patient. These directions typically include the dose amount, frequency, and sometimes duration of the medication being ordered. An example would be if a doctor wrote a prescription for Percocet-5 tablets. A typical sig for this medication could be "i-ii q4-6hrs."

To make the process of order entry more efficient, pharmacy software employs the use of sig codes when entering orders. **Sig codes** are programmed abbreviations for common sig instructions. This abbreviated entry requires fewer keystrokes to enter in, many times removing spaces, and therefore decreases the time it takes to enter an order. For example, rather than typing into the software "Take 1 tablet by mouth twice daily," a sig code could be "1TBID." This takes less time to type. This process can be expanded to cover specific drugs and sigs as well. If the standard drug used for ulcer prevention in a given facility is Prevacid 20 mg qd, a sig code could be programmed for PREV20 that would fill in all relevant fields. There is no universal sig code list; these are developed in house for the specific needs of the facility.

Warning Screens

An important aspect of medication order entry is warning screens and their function. **Warning screens** are pop-up windows that activate when certain criteria are met when entering orders (**Figure 11-3**). When a medication is entered for a patient, the pharmacy software screens it against the patient's other medications, conditions, allergies, and the like for safety.

Some warning screens that can activate include drug–drug interactions, toxicity warnings, duplicate therapy, and contraindications. Typically, the technician has the ability to bypass a warning screen and continue entering the order. This depends on the severity of the warning. In other instances, a pharmacist must review the warning screen and enter their initials in order to bypass it. The rules regarding bypass ability are controlled via settings within the pharmacy software, and can be adjusted according to facility policies.

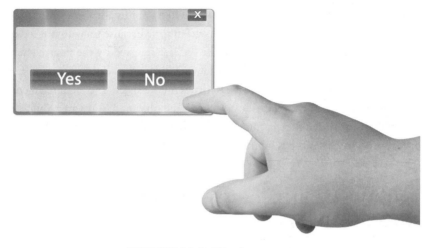

FIGURE 11-3 Warning screen.

© artiomp/Shutterstock, Inc.

TIPS AND TRICKS
To Bypass or Not to Bypass

Just because a warning screen is able to be bypassed does not mean that it always should be. Some warnings are not commonly that dangerous, and seem more like an annoying extra click most of the time. When first learning the process of order entry, however, it is important to notify the pharmacist of all warning screens encountered, and let them make the decision of what to bypass. If it is one that a technician has the ability to bypass, the technician should then ask why it can be bypassed, and also in what instances it should not be bypassed.

Order Sets

Standardization in a hospital is desired for many reasons. When procedures are standardized, there is less room for errors and an increase in efficiency. Medication orders can also be standardized. An **order set** is a programmed list of medications that can be selected during order entry. For example, there could be an order set for all patients being admitted to the intensive care unit in a given facility. The physician uses an order sheet with a preprinted list of medications.

The physician selects which drugs they would like to order for their patient, usually by checking a box. This saves the physician time because they do not have to write all of the orders by hand. When the order is received by the pharmacy, the technician can enter the name of the order set in the medication selection field. This would then pull up the same list of drugs on the sheet. The technician could then check the specific medications ordered. The pharmacy software would then input all of the ordered drugs at once. This saves the technician from having to enter every drug into the system individually.

ORDER SCANNING SOFTWARE AND EQUIPMENT

In the past, order sheets in a patient's chart had carbon copies attached to them. When a doctor wrote a medication order in the chart, there were at least three copies of it. One of those copies would be transferred to the pharmacy, much like a prescription in the retail setting. This would be accomplished by the nurse or maybe a CNA bringing down the order, or a technician making rounds to pick them up from nursing units. The process of receiving a medication order in the pharmacy has become almost entirely electronic in most hospital settings. As a result of this, it is necessary to understand the software and equipment used in the field for this process.

Benefits

There are many advantages to utilizing scanning software technology. It has had a significant impact on order processing in a hospital setting. The benefits to this type of equipment include the following:

- *Decreased turnaround time:* **Turnaround time** is a term for how long it takes from the point an order has been written until the medication is administered to the patient. With hardcopy delivery, this process could take more than an hour. With near instantaneous transmission of the order to the pharmacy, as well as ADC use, the turnaround time can be reduced to minutes.
- *Documentation:* Paper copies can be misplaced, and filing of documents can be time consuming as well as space consuming (**Figure 11-4**). Finding an order from last week would be a lengthy prospect, let alone an order from a month ago. With digital archiving, documents are

retrievable quickly and space concerns are negligible.

- *Legibility:* Medication orders are sometimes difficult to decipher. Scanning software has the ability to zoom in on scanned images and even adjust contrast in order to better translate the order for entry.

Scanning Equipment

Instead of having to pick up or deliver hard copies of medication orders, nurse stations in a facility are equipped with scanning devices that are connected to the pharmacy department. These devices can look like a fax machine or other document scanning devices (see **Figure 11-5**). When an order is written, either

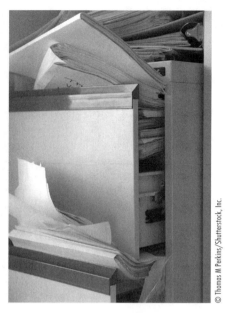

FIGURE 11-4 The pitfalls of paper records.

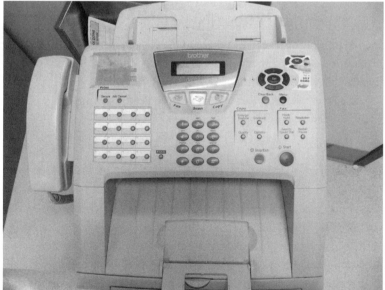

FIGURE 11-5 Devices such as these allow nurses to digitally scan orders to the pharmacy.

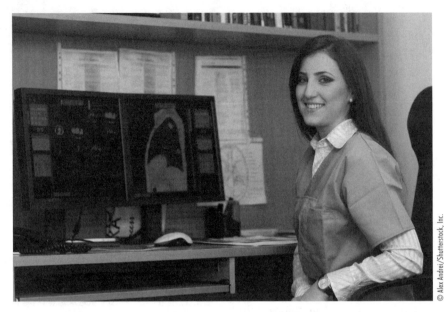

© Alex Andrei/Shutterstock, Inc.

FIGURE 11-6 Dual monitors allow for easier viewing of digitally scanned medication orders.

the nurse, charge nurse, or unit secretary may scan the order using this device, which then transmits the scanned image to the pharmacy.

In pharmacies with this type of technology, computers used for order entry will typically have two monitors (see **Figure 11-6**). One is to display the pharmacy management software, and the other is dedicated to displaying the scanned medication order for entry into the system.

SUMMARY

There is often a fear of having to learn a new computer program when working in a pharmacy. The idea is that it is going to be completely different from anything ever before encountered. In reality, most pharmacy software programs are highly similar—not necessarily in appearance or structure, but in functionality. By understanding the principles of what pharmacy software and peripheral devices are used for in the field, a new technician or trainee should have less difficulty adapting to any particular system. That lack of fear and increased willingness to learn will only improve the impression made by any student or trainee to their employers.

REVIEW QUESTIONS

1. What kinds of basic computer programs should be learned to navigate most pharmacy management systems?
2. List three tasks that can be performed by a technician using pharmacy management software.
3. What steps in the order entry process are at risk for error? Why?
4. Name three reasons a warning screen could pop up during order entry operations.
5. Define turnaround time. Why is this important in terms of patient care?
6. What are some benefits of order scanning equipment and software?
7. What would be a reason the pharmacy tech would credit medications back to the patient's profile? Why is it such an important task?

CHAPTER 12

Automation Software and Peripherals

LEARNING OBJECTIVES

Upon completion of this chapter, you will be able to

1. Describe the connections between a main console and ADC technology
2. Define the override process and its importance with ADC operations
3. Recognize various peripheral devices and their use with ADC technology

KEY TERMS

Connectivity	Override
Critical override	

INTRODUCTION

Automation technology for medication dispensing has changed the face of pharmacy operations in the health system setting. Whether it is in the form of an automated dispensing cabinet (ADC) or a robotic device, there must be a means for

Table 12-1 Dispensing Systems

Anesthesia ADC Systems	ADC Systems	Robotic Systems
CareFusion Pyxis Anesthesia System	ABTG MedSelect Rx Cabinets	McKesson Robot-Rx
McKesson Anesthesia-Rx	CareFusion Pyxis MedStation System	Swisslog PillPick
Omnicell Anesthesia Workstation	Cerner RxStation	
	McKesson AcuDose-Rx	
	Metro MedDispense	
	Omnicell OmniRx	

the technician to interact with it. This is where hardware and peripherals come into play. By understanding how some of these peripheral devices and hardware interact, it is possible for a technician to anticipate challenges as well as opportunities to improve their operation.

In terms of types of technology in use in the field, it is good to be familiar with the major systems on the market. Although made by different companies, functionality is similar in regards to medication dispensing activities. Knowing the names of systems is part of knowing the jargon of the industry. When going to buy a car, a person typically knows the makes and models of vehicles they are interested in. It would be safe to assume that a technician looking to apply for a job would want to be familiar with the types of automation they could be working with. See **Table 12-1** for a list of different automation systems. More information about a particular system can be found at each company's website.

MAIN CONSOLE

There is a main computer console located in the pharmacy that is the control hub for every ADC in the facility. Often called simply "the main," or even "the brain," this computer is connected to every ADC as well as to the pharmacy management software (**Figure 12-1**). The pharmacy management software transfers patient information to the console, as well as the medication orders that have been entered into them. This main console can also retrieve data from ADCs, including inventories, access records, and locations of different medications.

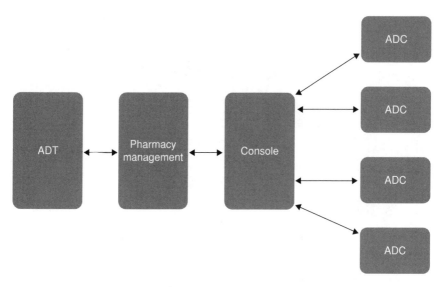

FIGURE 12-1 Information transfer between main console and ADCs in a hospital setting.

The software for ADC technology follows the same principles as traditional Windows applications, with drop-down menus at the top of the window for different operations or procedures. Depending on the level of access of the user, different features may or may not be accessible.

CONNECTIVITY

Connectivity deals with the ability of different computer systems and devices to communicate with one another. For automation, there are concepts and equipment to examine when learning about how the main console communicates with the pharmacy management software as well as the ADC cabinets. All of these devices are networked together using standard Ethernet cables to allow them to transmit data, much like most home Internet setups (**Figure 12-2**). These cables are connected through a network hub, which funnels input and output information to the main console (**Figure 12-3**).

As information is transferred between the main console and respective ADCs, or between the pharmacy management system and main console, the database will refresh itself to reflect the most recent communications between devices. The interval of the communication refresh time on the main console can be set by

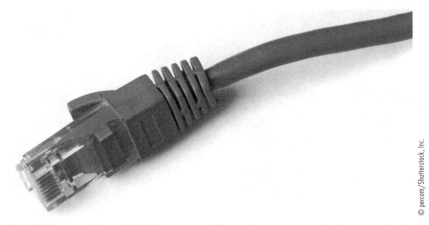

© percom/Shutterstock, Inc.

FIGURE 12-2 A standard ethernet cord for information transfer between devices.

the user, and can also be can manually initiated. One aspect of the main console software is the ability to review the communication logs for each ADC in the facility. This option is useful to determine the connectivity of a particular machine. For example, a nurse may call the pharmacy to notify a technician that the drugs that were entered for her patient are not showing up on the patient's profile on a particular ADC. After confirming that the medication was in fact entered in

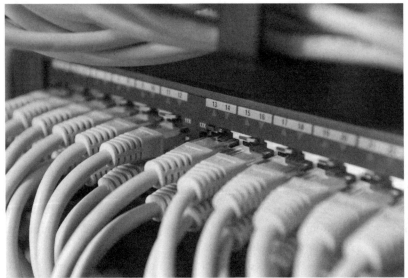

© Kjetil Kolbjornsrud/Shutterstock, Inc.

FIGURE 12-3 Network hubs allow the connection of multiple
devices to a single network or server.

the patient profile and is showing up on the main console, the next step would be to check the communication log for that particular ADC. If the log showed no updates for an extended period of time, it would most likely be the reason why that information is not available to the nurse. The order data is not being transmitted to the ADC. At that point the technician could try to manually initiate a refresh, and if that did not solve the problem, take further action with technical support.

OVERRIDES

Sometimes a medication must be given before the order for it has been reviewed by a pharmacist and entered into the patient's profile. If a nurse wishes to remove a drug from the ADC in this fashion, the process is called an **override**. It is called this because the nurse or doctor is overriding the system to access the medication. The situations that call for a medication override are stat orders and cases in which harm would come to the patient if they did not receive the drug immediately. All overrides are documented by the ADC. It may be a technician's responsibility to review override logs on a scheduled basis to determine if they are legitimate overrides, or to follow up to see if an order has been written postadministration.

Critical Override

At times there can be a break in communications between the pharmacy management software and the main console. When this happens, no new medication orders are able to be transmitted to *any* of the ADCs in the facility. At this point there is an option to place all ADCs into a setting commonly called **critical override**. When cabinets are in critical override, all medications are able to be overridden, essentially allowing nursing to take out whatever medication they need when they need it. There is usually a policy in the hospital manual on the steps taken when initiating a critical override. This can include an announcement on the overhead system alerting nurses that a critical override has been initiated. This helps limit the number of additional phone calls to the pharmacy department.

HANDHELD SCANNER DEVICES AND APPLICATIONS

Batch refill reports originally printed out on paper in the pharmacy. This is still done in many facilities; however, there is new technology that is in use if utilizing CareFusion Pyxis brand ADC technology. This technology removes the need for paper batch reports. It is called Pyxis PARx. This addition to ADC technology further enhances safety and accuracy in the medication pulling process. Medication pulling is one of the first areas where a medication error can be made by a technician. If a technician pulls the wrong medication or the wrong dose of that medication, for example, and a pharmacist does not catch the mistake, it could be loaded incorrectly into the ADC. This risk is minimized greatly by the PARx system through the use of barcode scanning technology. The medication is verified by scanning its barcode rather than the traditional visual verification. There are several additional pieces of equipment that the technician utilizes with the PARx system:

- *Handheld scanner:* This device is similar to others used to order stock for a company. Instead of a paper refill report, the list is wirelessly uploaded to the scanner and displayed for the technician. It has a laser scanner for barcode scanning purposes. The technician would go to the bin holding the medication displayed on the scanner, and then scan the barcode printed on the packaging. This verifies correct selection. If the wrong medication was selected, the scanner would notify the technician.
- *Label printer:* This device is wirelessly connected to the handheld scanner. Once a medication is scanned and pulled, the label printer generates a label, also with a barcode printed on it. This label is affixed to the plastic sealable bag that the pulled medication is placed in. This will be used for verification.
- *Check station:* This device is a computer workstation and is used to aid the pharmacist or other technician in verification of the batch refill. It also has a barcode scanner. The person performing the verification scans the label on the plastic sealable bag and visually checks the medication stored within it. After this process has occurred, delivery to the ADC for refilling may proceed.

SUMMARY

There are many components and equipment that are used with automation technology in order to operate ADCs effectively. The main console controls all ADCs, and the mechanisms with which it does so must be understood. There are different settings and actions that can be used in situations when communication or network connection issues arise. An ancillary device such as PARx increases the safety of ADC refill operations.

REVIEW QUESTIONS

1. What types of automation are used in local hospitals in the area? Are they brands discussed in this chapter?
2. Explain the relationship between pharmacy management and ADC networks. How do they communicate?
3. What is connectivity, and how does it affect ADC interfaces?
4. When is a critical override necessary in a hospital setting?
5. Name two situations in which a nurse may need to override a medication.
6. What is the benefit of technology such as the PARx system in medication filling for ADCs?

Repackaging Technology

INTRODUCTION

Oral medications in a health system setting are dispensed in unit dose packages. Unit dose packaging decreases waste and increases the efficiency and accuracy of medication dispensing activities. The average length of stay for a patient in a health system is 3 to 5 days. Medications are dispensed for 24 hours at a time. It would not be the wisest use of manpower and supplies to dispense medication using the community setting model. Using an amber vial and counting tray to dispense only two pills would be counterproductive (**Figure 13-1**).

PILL AND CAPSULE REPACKAGING

Manufacturers produce a majority of their medications in both bulk and unit dose packaging. Remember that a **unit dose** is a medication packaged individually per pill or capsule (see **Figure 13-2**). **Bulk** packaging is a bottle of pills or capsules, typically in quantities of 30, 50, 100, 1,000, and so on (see **Figure 13-3**).

Some medications are not available from the manufacturer in a unit dose form. When a bulk container for a medication is received in a health system pharmacy,

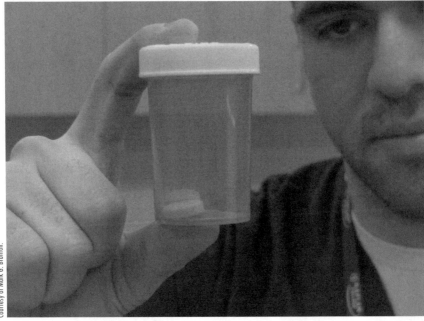

Courtesy of Mark G. Brunton.

FIGURE 13-1 A whole amber vial for 2 pills? Really?

it is the job of the pharmacy technician to put it into a unit dose package. This process is known as **repackaging**.

Repackaging Automation

In the past, when medications needed to be repackaged, it was done entirely by hand. A technician would place the medication one at a time into a sheet of unit dose containers, and then seal them with labeled backing at the end. Although this method may still be in use in certain settings, the more common way is to utilize a repackaging

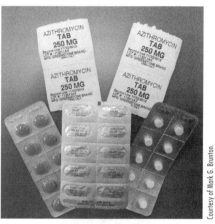

FIGURE 13-2 Examples of unit dose packaging.

machine to automate the process. A repackaging machine greatly increases the number of medications that can be unit dosed in a given time period versus repackaging by hand.

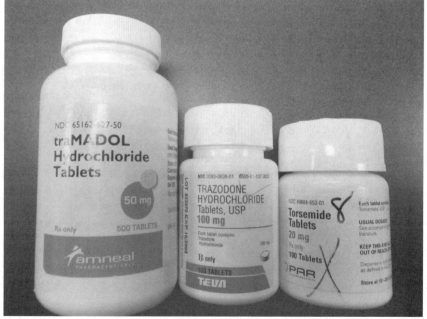

FIGURE 13-3 Examples of bulk packaging.

Anatomy of a Repackaging Machine

The following is a breakdown of components for a typical repackaging machine. As with other forms of technology, there may be variations depending on brand, but overall functionality remains the same. Using **Figure 13-4** as a reference, the following are the major components of a repacking machine:

1. *Thermal paper roll:* This provides the back to the unit dose package, with medication information printed on it.
2. *Controller module:* This unit communicates with the computer used for repackaging software as well as the printer module. The buttons on this device are used to start the repackager when ready, as well as to clear any data between different medication repackaging procedures.
3. *Thermal printer:* This device prints the pertinent information onto the thermal paper backing. This can include drug name, strength, dose form, manufacturer, expiration date, barcode identifier, and so on.

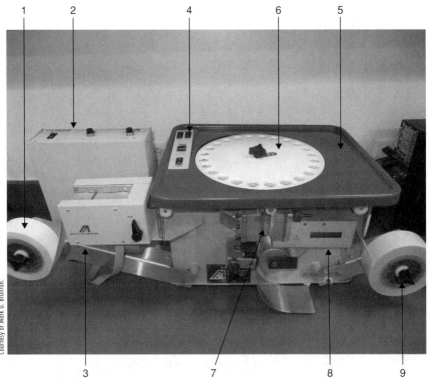

Courtesy of Mark G. Brunton.

FIGURE 13-4 Anatomy of a repackaging machine.

4. *Power switches:* These turn on the heating element of the machine, as well as the feed disk engine.

5. *Loading tray:* This is where medication is placed by the technician during operation of the machine.

6. *Feed disk:* This is what places the medication into the unit dose packaging.

7. *Heating element:* This mechanism presses together to heat seal the clear front and paper backing of the dispensing rolls.

8. *Temperature indicator:* Displays the current temperature of the heating element.

9. *Clear plastic roll:* This provides the front of the unit dose package. It is transparent in order to allow visual verification of correct medication once repackaging is complete.

Repackaging Procedure

The process to repackage medications is fairly straightforward. The steps used are identical regardless of the type of pill or capsule being packaged. One of the quickest ways to learn how to operate the machine is to repackage several medications consecutively to become comfortable with the procedure.

The following lists the basic steps for how to repackage a medication using a repackaging machine:

1. *Clean loading tray:* This task is accomplished with 70% isopropyl alcohol, in exactly the same fashion as cleaning a pill counting tray (**Figure 13-5**).

2. *Turn on the device:* This will turn on the heating element, a key step. The digital temperature display will indicate when it is at a sufficient heat level to seal the packaging around the medication. This heating-up phase can take several minutes, so it is best to initiate it early in the process.

3. *Initialize computer software:* This is where you will control what the machine will print when you begin the repackaging process.

4. *Program the label:* Once the software is initialized, the information for specific medication labeling may be input into the computer to be transferred to the control box and machine.

5. *Load medications:* Empty the desired quantity of medications to be repackaged onto the loading tray (**Figure 13-6**). Note that if repackaging large quantities of a medication, it may be necessary to repeat this process more than once, because all of the pills or capsules may not fit on the loading tray at one time.

6. *Start the machine:* The feed disk will begin to rotate at a controlled pace, dropping the medication between the thermal paper and clear plastic as

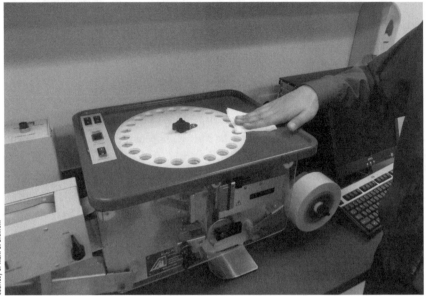

Courtesy of Mark G. Brunton.

FIGURE 13-5 Cleaning a repackaging machine.

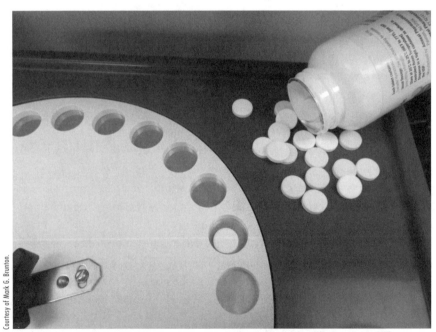

Courtesy of Mark G. Brunton.

FIGURE 13-6 Loading medications on a repackaging machine.

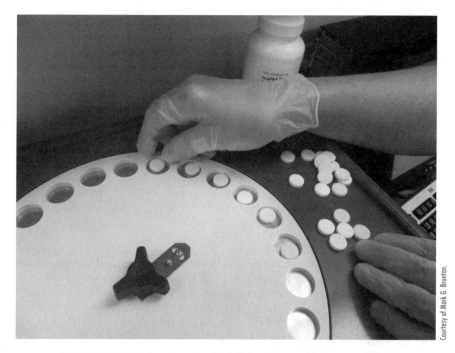

Courtesy of Mark G. Brunton.

FIGURE 13-7 Loading the feed disk of a repackaging machine.

it is sealed together by the heating element. As this occurs, the technician refills the loading wheel with more pills or capsules as it rotates, much like a revolving door–type mechanism (**Figure 13-7**).

7. *Final steps:* After completion of the repackaging procedure, the technician will prepare the completed medications as well as proper documentation to give to the pharmacist for final verification. A repackaged medication can never be placed into stock for dispensing until the pharmacist has verified the accuracy of the procedure. (Note that some facilities are now using the tech-check-tech system for this activity.)

Documentation and Labeling

When a medication is repackaged, it is not going directly to a patient but rather onto the shelf to be dispensed later. Regardless, the medication is changing containers, from a bulk to a unit dose container. Because of this transfer, certain rules must be followed and documentation must occur. All of the pertinent information on the original manufacturer's container must be recorded to be able to track the medication after it has changed containers. Traditionally this task could be recorded on a **repackaging control log**, which was recorded by hand. With the advent of repackaging automation, the software that controls the machine also can generate a repackaging log printout after operations are completed.

Several key pieces of information need to be transferred to the unit dose packaging from the bulk container. These include the following:

- Drug name
- Drug strength
- Drug dosage form
- Drug manufacturer
- Lot number
- Expiration date

These items are required, but additional information may be needed as prescribed by the internal policies and procedures of a given facility.

Completion and Verification

Upon completion of repackaging procedures, a technician should clean the machine, making sure there is no leftover medication residue and general trash accumulated during the procedure. It is also very important to *turn the machine off* when not in use. This is a very easy step to forget to do, and happens more often than one would expect. If a repackaging machine is left on for an extended period of time, it can lead to damage of the heating element on the device, requiring service or replacement.

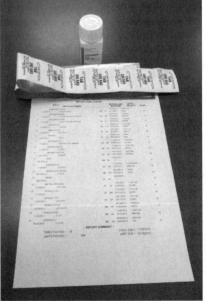

The pharmacist needs several items in order to verify a completed repackaging procedure (**Figure 13-8**). These include:

- The repackaged medication
- The original bulk container
- Repackaging log documentation

After the pharmacist has verified the medication, it can be placed into stock in the pharmacy, and the documentation filed in the appropriate location.

FIGURE 13-8 Repackaging setup for verification.

Courtesy of Mark G. Brunton.

ORAL LIQUID REPACKAGING

As with pills and capsules, oral liquids may or may not be available in a unit dosed form from the manufacturer (**Figure 13-9**). If not available, it is again the technician's responsibility to repackage the medication for use.

There are some oral liquid repackaging machines available for use in the pharmacy, but these are less prevalent than the pill and capsule versions. More often, oral liquids are still repackaged by hand. The procedure differs depending on the unit dose container utilized in the repackaging operation. The following sections describe some of the most common oral liquid unit dose containers. Note that documentation and verification practices are the same as with other repackaging processes.

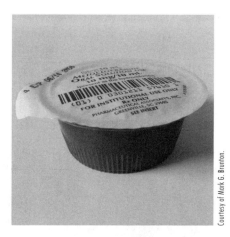

FIGURE 13-9 An example of a manufacturer-prepared unit dose oral liquid medication.

Courtesy of Mark G. Brunton.

Dose Cups

Dose cups are small containers that can hold volumes from 5 ml to 45 ml, as necessary, for different types of medications. They have a peel-away covering and are able to be administered directly from the container, rather than having to be poured into a dosing cup. They generally come packaged in trays of 30, and can be filled relatively quickly. The steps for repackaging in this form are as follows:

1. *Prepare the medication to be repackaged:* There are various methods for preparing the medication. One common practice is to pour the amount into a glass mortar, and utilize a large volume syringe, such as 60 ml, to transfer the liquid to the dose cups (**Figure 13-10**).

2. *Flip the tray over:* Note that there is a hole in the bottom of each dose cup (**Figure 13-11**). This is where the oral liquid will be transferred.

3. *Transfer liquid:* A large volume syringe should have the ability to fill several dose cups without refilling, depending on dose size (**Figure 13-12**).

4. *Seal dose cups:* The hole in the bottom of the dose cup is sealed with a plastic sphere, similar in shape to an Airsoft BB round. These are pushed into the hole until held in place by friction, either by hand or with the use of a handheld device that holds the BBs.

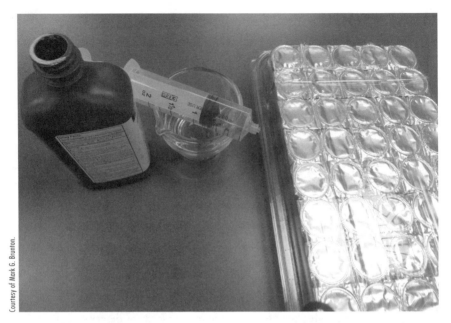

FIGURE 13-10 Medication preparation for liquid unit dose repackaging.

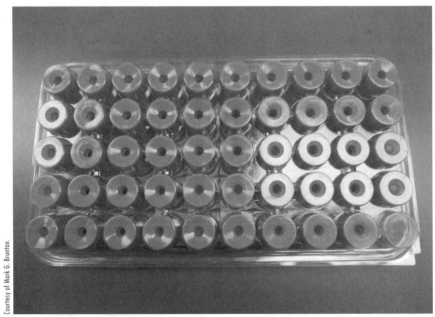

FIGURE 13-11 Flip tray over.

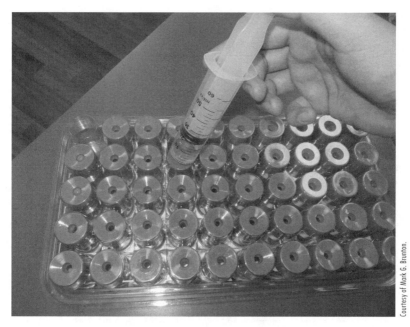

Courtesy of Mark G. Brunton.

FIGURE 13-12 Oral liquid transfer to dose cups.

5. *Label:* Flip the tray back over, and affix proper labels to the tops of the dose cups (**Figure 13-13**).

6. *Verify:* Prepare dose cups, original bulk container, and appropriate documentation for pharmacist approval.

Oral Syringes

An **oral syringe** is another vehicle for administering oral liquid medication to a patient. Oral syringes may be used instead of dose cups for several reasons. The first is for uncooperative or unconscious patients. The oral liquid can be injected into a nasogastric tube to deliver the medication. Oral syringes are also widely used for infants who cannot swallow pills or capsules.

There are several specific differences between an IV syringe and an oral syringe (**Figure 13-14**). These differences

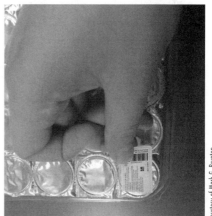

Courtesy of Mark G. Brunton.

FIGURE 13-13 Labeling of dose cups.

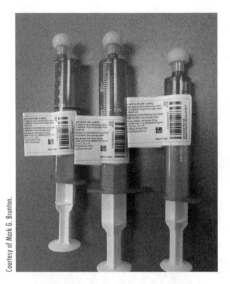

Courtesy of Mark G. Brunton.

FIGURE 13-14 Examples of oral syringes.

are very important to prevent accidental injection of an oral medication into an IV line. This mistake has happened in the hospital setting. A pharmacy technician should never put an oral medication into an IV syringe. Oral syringes are usually amber colored, much like other oral medication containers, to protect light-sensitive medications. They are also clearly labeled with the words "For oral use only." Oral syringes also are designed with a tip shape that prevents it from attaching or remaining attached to any IV equipment.

The standard steps for repackaging a bulk oral medication into an oral syringe are as follows:

1. *Adapter attachment:* The most efficient means to withdraw an oral medication from the bulk container is to attach a syringe adapter to its opening. This adapter allows an oral syringe to be attached to the bulk container in order to manipulate fluid transfer, much like an IV fluid transfer.

2. *Fluid withdrawal:* While holding the bulk container inverted in one hand, the required volume of medication is withdrawn into the oral syringe with the other hand (**Figure 13-15**).

3. *Capping the syringe:* Placing a cap onto the oral syringe involves pressing the tip of the syringe firmly into the cap to seal the medication for dispensing (**Figure 13-16**).

4. *Labeling:* Labels are attached to an oral syringe using the flag technique. Both ends of the label are attached to the barrel of the syringe, with the rest of the label being pinched together, essentially creating a tiny flag out of the label (**Figure 13-17**).

Courtesy of Mark G. Brunton.

FIGURE 13-15 Fluid withdrawal.

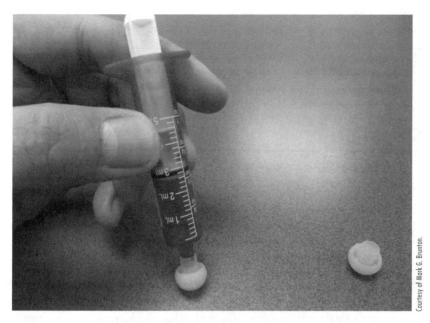

Courtesy of Mark G. Brunton.

FIGURE 13-16 Capping an oral syringe.

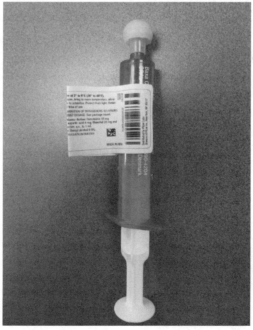

Courtesy of Mark G. Brunton.

FIGURE 13-17 Oral syringe labeling.

> Do not cover the measurements on a syringe when labeling.

5. *Verification:* Prepare oral syringes, original bulk container, and appropriate documentation for pharmacist approval.

SUMMARY

Unit dosed medications are an essential element of medication dispensing in a health system setting. When a manufacturer of a particular medication does not provide a unit dose form of packaging, it is the responsibility of the pharmacy technician to repackage it into a suitable unit dose.

Oral medications such as pills, capsules, and liquids can all be unit dosed by a pharmacy technician. In many cases, there are forms of automation that can help facilitate these procedures. It is very important to follow established guidelines and documentation requirements when taking any medication and transferring it from one container to another. This is to ensure the highest degree of medication safety for the patient.

REVIEW QUESTIONS

1. Why are unit dosed medications necessary in a hospital setting?
2. What are the risks, if any, of repackaging operations?
3. List four pieces of information that must be printed on a repackaged medication.
4. What is the importance of documentation for repackaging operations?
5. What are some uses for oral syringes in the hospital setting?

IV Room Technology

KEY TERMS

Calibration

Critical site

First air

High efficiency particulate air (HEPA)

Pass-through

Precipitation

Total parenteral nutrition (TPN)

INTRODUCTION

In addition to the specific devices used in the manipulations of sterile products such as syringes, needles, and the like, there are other pieces of equipment that are used for IV compounding operations. This chapter will describe these devices, as well as standard procedures for maintenance and quality assurance procedures relating to them. **Figure 14-1** illustrates a technician working in a horizontal laminar flow hood, a common piece of equipment used when making sterile products.

HORIZONTAL LAMINAR AIRFLOW WORKBENCHES

Also abbreviated as LAFW, the workbench is often called just "the hood." This is the physical area where IV preparations are actually compounded. It consists of a stainless steel work surface for compounding with ultraclean air being blown across the workspace from a vent. The blowing air keeps the area surrounding the IV free of contamination from airborne particles. The air being blown across the workspace is filtered through two air filters. The first is a large particulate filter, much like the ones used for air conditioning and heating in houses. The second is a **high efficiency particulate air (HEPA)** filter. This filter removes almost all potential contaminants from the air being pushed across the work surface. This adds another layer of protection in conjunction with proper aseptic technique.

When working in this type of environment, aseptic manipulations must follow certain guidelines for the workbench to be effective. IVs must be compounded at least 6 inches inside the workbench at all times in order to ensure maximum sterility (**Figure 14-2**).

The orientation of objects within the workspace, including hand placement, must also be very specific when dealing with horizontal airflow. A common term used when discussing this principle is **first air**, which is the object that

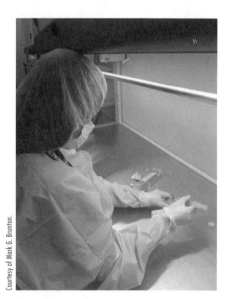

Courtesy of Mark G. Brunton.

FIGURE 14-1 An IV technician in a hospital setting.

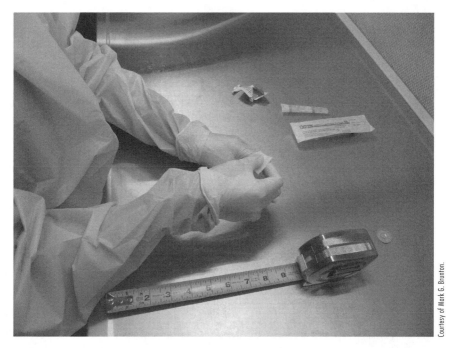

Courtesy of Mark G. Brunton.

FIGURE 14-2 Six inches inside an LAFW. Note that the tape measure is used merely to illustrate distance, but would never be in a laminar flow hood under actual work conditions.

first comes into contact with air from the HEPA filter. This air is free from contaminants, and therefore should have direct access to critical sites. **Critical sites** are any area where direct contact with the medication or IV solution occurs. Typically these are the areas that are punctured with a needle.

BARRIER ISOLATORS

Also known as a glovebox, this workbench is completely enclosed and has armholes with attached gloves to access the work surface (**Figure 14-3**). A technician reaches their hands into the arms to begin IV compounding procedures. Materials for the compounding process are passed into the work area via an airlock called a **pass-through** in order to maintain sterility. This type of workbench is becoming more popular in IV rooms because it satisfies many requirements of United States Pharmacopeia Chapter 797 (USP 797) without the need to remodel or reconfigure the entire IV room (Wagner, 2012). One challenge with this workbench is that it can slow down IV compounding processes slightly.

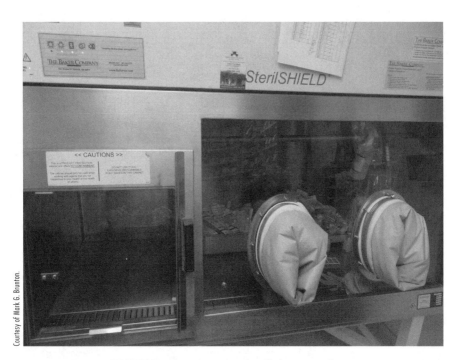

Courtesy of Mark G. Brunton.

FIGURE 14-3 An example of a barrier isolator.

BIOLOGICAL SAFETY CABINETS

In this type of workbench, airflow is directed from the top of the hood downward. This mechanism is similar to the air curtains seen at supermarkets. There is also a guard panel in the front, which protects the technician during compounding operations. Due to the protective capabilities of this workbench, it is primarily used for compounding hazardous materials such as chemotherapeutic agents. This type of workbench may also be referred to as a class II biological safety cabinet, a vertical flow hood, or a chemo hood.

COMPOUNDING DEVICES

Several devices used in the IV room automate certain processes, making them more accurate and efficient. This can make a technician's workflow easier to manage. Most involve transferring fluid more effectively. An example would be an IV

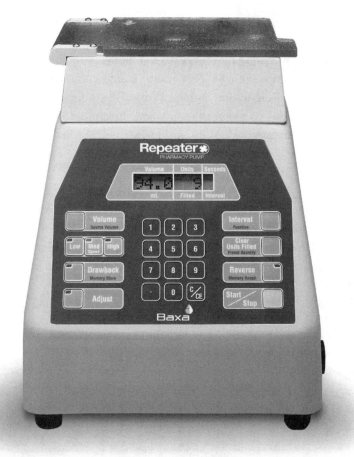

Courtesy of Baxter International, Inc.

FIGURE 14-4 Example of an IV compounding pump.

fluid compounding pump (see **Figure 14-4**). This device transfers fluids from one container to another. It can be from a large volume IV bag to a smaller one, or into prefilled syringes. Its operation can be controlled by a foot pedal, allowing for hands-free operation. The technician's role with this device would be to calibrate it to pump the correct amount of fluid, as well as to replace the plastic tubing that is used in its operation.

TPN Compounder

Total parenteral nutrition (TPN) is a very specialized form of IV preparation that provides all of the nutritional needs for a patient via the IV route. TPN is used when a patient cannot receive food through the gastrointestinal route. Each TPN dose is specifically formulated for an individual patient. It has numerous ingredients, and preparing one can take a significant amount of time. The original process for compounding a TPN was by hand, with the technician mixing upwards of 24 medications into a single IV bag. The order of compounding was very specific in order to prevent precipitation. **Precipitation** in IV solutions is when two or more medications do not mix with each other. This can produce cloudiness in the solution or crystallization, which can harm a patient rather than help them.

In order to streamline this process, the use of a TPN compounder has become common practice (see **Figure 14-5**). This device has multiple plastic tubing lines that connect via spike adapters to the numerous ingredients used in a TPN. There are also ports for syringes filled with additional ingredients. These tubes are all directed to one port connected to an empty IV bag. The

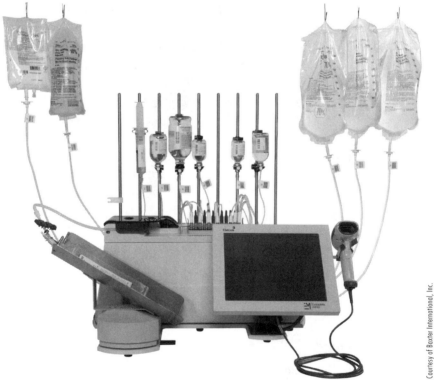

FIGURE 14-5 Example of a TPN compounder.

Courtesy of Baxter International, Inc.

machine is programmed with a specific patient's TPN order. The compounder then proceeds to withdraw the appropriate drugs and mix them into one bag. The technician's role with this device is to calibrate it daily to ensure accuracy and to replace medications that are used up during the compounding process. Every line of tubing has a barcode label attached to it, and the patient's order is barcoded as well. This ensures accurate replacement of medication and proper patient identification. The automation of this process frees up time for the technician to work on other IV orders during TPN compounding operations (Osteen, 2011).

Robotics is a growing field for IV automation, with a robot currently on the market that can make an entire IV preparation from beginning to end (see **Figure 14-6**). It is currently most often used for the preparation of chemotherapeutic agents. The technician's role is not eliminated when working with this machine, but rather changed by it. The technician becomes responsible for loading the necessary medications and fluids into the robot for compounding, calibration, troubleshooting, and other duties. The only current IV robot device in the United States is the IntelliFill robot made by Baxter.

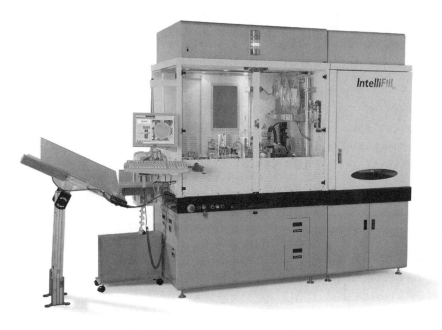

Courtesy of Baxter International, Inc.

FIGURE 14-6 Example of an IV robot.

IN THE FIELD
Fear of Change and Technology

Whenever there is new technology that can do a task normally delegated to a pharmacy technician, there is an element of fear. "What if they don't need me anymore?" "Are they going to cut staff?" "This thing is going to take my job!" These are some of the thoughts that can go through your head, but there is another perspective to view it from. First, these are the same thoughts that occurred to pharmacists when the pharmacy technician position was created. And there are still pharmacists. But what happened to their roles and responsibilities? They expanded and redefined the scope of their practice, focusing more on patient care and medication therapy. This is one tactic to consider when confronted with changes in technology. Explore new areas of work that a technician can perform. Remember, if the law doesn't specifically state that a pharmacist has to do an activity, that means a *pharmacy technician* can perform that task.

Another strategy is to master the new technology. There will always be bugs to work out with any new system, and no one else in the pharmacy knows how this system or technology works either. This is your chance to learn everything you can about it. Learn how to maintain, calibrate, and troubleshoot it. Learn how to optimize it, or make it run better. In that case, if there is a reduction in workforce, it is not you that they will choose to let go. People who refuse to learn a new system or technology soon find they are obsolete in the new order of things, and then become expendable.

MAINTENANCE AND QUALITY CONTROL

All devices in the pharmacy that deal with medications must be properly cleaned and maintained. The quality of sterile preparations must be controlled and kept at the level needed to ensure safe treatment for the patient. Poorly maintained or seldom cleaned equipment can lead to infection and possibly even death as a result of contaminated sterile products. The following sections discuss the concepts involved with proper maintenance and quality control. A technician can expect to perform these actions if working in an IV room setting.

Calibration

Calibration involves comparing a device's stated measurement against another scale of measure to determine accuracy. In the case of IV compounding and TPN compounding devices, the common method of calibration is to use a digital scale (see **Figure 14-7**). An amount of sterile water pumped from the device is weighed to check that it is pumping correctly. One milliliter of water is equal to 1 gram. So if a technician programs the pump to dispense 50 ml, the weight of the water should be 50 grams.

Typically if the numbers are not equal, the technician would enter the discrepancy into the pump and it would attempt to autocorrect for the error. The weight calibration check may have to be done several times until the pump is working accurately and calibration has been accomplished.

Cleaning

In general, all work surfaces in an IV room should be cleaned with 70% isopropyl alcohol to help ensure sterility. Different equipment will have their own

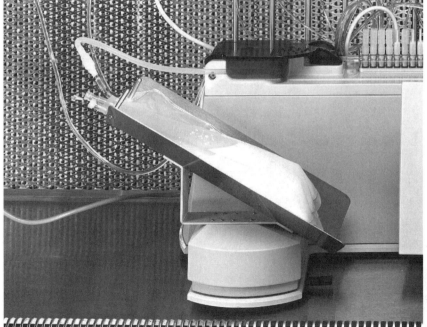

Courtesy of Baxter International, Inc.

FIGURE 14-7 By weighing an amount of liquid dispensed, calibrations can be made to the compounder.

recommendations on cleaning technique and schedule from their manufacturer. Typically, surface cleaning of devices should be taking place very regularly, with scheduled periods to do a thorough deep cleaning, usually involving a tear down of the machine (**Figure 14-8**). These guidelines will be in the manual for the equipment in question.

Documentation

Activities that have to be done on a regular basis in the IV room, such as those listed in the previous sections, must be documented in order to ensure compliance. These activities will have log sheets that have to be filled out to prove that, for example, a piece of equipment was cleaned at least four times every day.

The Joint Commission takes a close look at quality control logs in an IV room to make sure that all preparations are being made in a clean environment and that the measurements have been consistently accurate. If a hospital's IV room logs have not been completed properly or are inconsistent, that would be a potential infraction during a Joint Commission inspection.

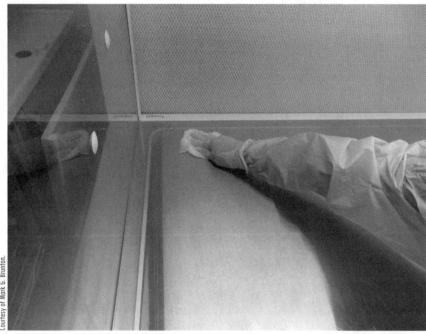

Courtesy of Mark G. Brunton.

FIGURE 14-8 IV equipment cleaning.

SUMMARY

There is more to making a proper IV than knowing how to use a syringe and being good at calculations. A wide variety of equipment and devices are used daily to assist the technician in completing their duties. The care and maintenance of these machines lies with the technician. Learning how to calibrate, clean, and document these activities is part of being a pharmacy technician in the IV room setting.

REVIEW QUESTIONS

1. Compare and contrast the strengths and weaknesses of different work areas used to compound IVs. Is one better than the others? Why or why not?
2. Why does a technician need to protect themselves when preparing chemotherapeutic agents?
3. Which device(s) would adequately protect a technician when preparing hazardous agents?
4. Why are calibrations important for IV compounding devices?
5. Explain the need for documentation of activities in an IV room.

REFERENCES

Osteen, R. (2011). Automating the in-house compounding process. *Pharmacy Purchasing and Products, 8*(7), 6. Retrieved from http://www.pppmag.com/article/922/July_2011/Automating_the_Inhouse_Compounding_Process/?TPN

Wagner, J. (2012). Assessing isolators for compounding operations. *Pharmacy Purchasing and Products, 9*(11), 42. Retrieved from http://www.pppmag.com/article/1221/November_2012/Assessing_Isolators_for_Compounding_Operations/?sterile compounding

Get Set for Your Career

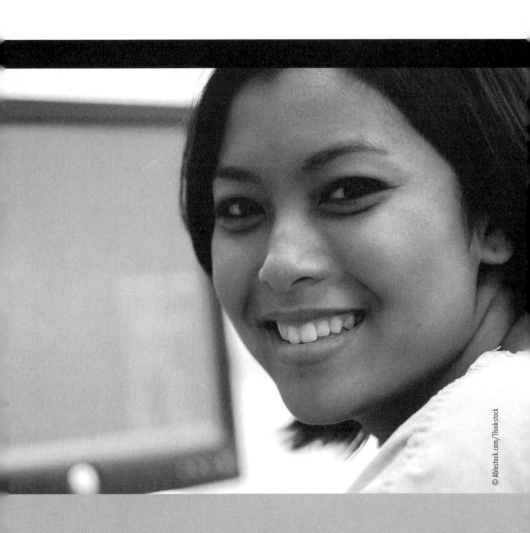

CHAPTER 15

Credentials

LEARNING OBJECTIVES

Upon completion of this chapter, you will be able to

1. Understand requirements for licensing, registration, and certification
2. Explain continuing education and requirements for state and national license renewal
3. Discuss the nature of professional organizations for pharmacy technicians and their importance to career development

KEY TERMS

Accreditation Council for Pharmacy Education (ACPE)

American Society of Health-System Pharmacists (ASHP)

Board of pharmacy

Certification

Certified Pharmacy Technician (CPhT)

Continuing education (CE)

Credentials

National Association of Boards of Pharmacy (NABP)

Professional organization

Reciprocity

INTRODUCTION

The definition of **credentials** is "a qualification, achievement, personal quality, etc., used to indicate suitability for something"(Credential, n.d.). With that definition in mind, all of the items discussed in this chapter indicate the suitability of a technician to be hired in a pharmacy. Some items are optional, whereas others are mandatory. Maintenance of necessary credentials not only will secure an opportunity for employment, but also is a requirement for continued employment.

LICENSES, REGISTRATIONS, AND CERTIFICATIONS

The laws that define the nature of a pharmacy technician's role vary from state to state. The terminology and requirements vary as well. In most states the term *licensed pharmacy technician* is used to indicate the ability to work in that state, regardless of whether the state actually licenses or registers its technicians. It is good to understand the different terms, with the understanding that often they are used interchangeably. As long as the requirements are understood and met in the state one is trying to work in, there should be no significant challenges to acquiring said licensure or registration. For simplicity, the term *license* will be used in this chapter.

There are some general items that are used in almost every state in regards to pharmacy technician applicants. States require a fee to be paid when applying to work in that state. The fee varies anywhere from $40 to more than $100. Some states will require national certification as well, or list it as one potential criterion, among several, that have to be met. Many states will also require as a potential criterion that an applicant have received training from a board-approved technician training program. The definition of this training program will again vary from state to state. It may include vocational training institutions, community college programs, or pharmacy in-house training programs. In order to know the requirements to work as a pharmacy technician in a given state, the specific state's board of pharmacy must be consulted. A **board of pharmacy** is the organization that handles the regulatory requirements for pharmacy in a state. The board's website will contain a section that addresses pharmacy technician requirements. These requirements will be either on the application itself or under a designated area of the webpage. The following is an example of requirements for licensure from the Nevada State Board of Pharmacy (Nevada State Board of Pharmacy, n.d.):

- Copy of certificate of completion of pharmaceutical technician program approved by the board.

- If you have a certificate from the Pharmacy Technician Certification Board (PTCB) or National Tech Exam (ICPT), you will be required to work in Nevada as a registered pharmaceutical technician in training for 500 hours. Please download the application for a pharmaceutical technician in training. If you send in a pharmacy technician application with PTCB or ICPT only, the application and fee will be returned.

You must include ONE of the following with the application:

- Copy of current registration or on-line verification from state in which you are currently registered as a pharmaceutical technician. Your license in the other state must be current to use for licensure in Nevada.
- Copy of a certificate from an ASHP approved pharmacy technician school. We only accept pharmacy technician schools that are ASHP (American Society of Health Pharmacists) approved. If your school is ASHP approved, the information will be included on your certificate from the school.

To find a particular board of pharmacy, one can simply search using a preferred search engine by entering the state's name and board of pharmacy. Another resource to find a board website is to go to the website for the **National Association of Boards of Pharmacy (NABP)**. This organization guides all of the boards of pharmacy. Its website contains a link to every state board of pharmacy. It also has additional pertinent information regarding pharmacy technician practice (National Association of Boards of Pharmacy, n.d.b.).

State Licensure

If a state officially *licenses* its technicians, certain criteria are required in order to use the term *licensed*. Much like a driver's license, one of the requirements is a test of some sort that has to be passed before licensure is granted. In Utah, for example, a technician applicant must complete and submit a Laws and Rules examination as well as national certification, pay a fee, and provide proof of either work experience or approved training.

State Registration

If a state *registers* its technicians, the criteria are generally less stringent than for states who license. Registration means literally that a pharmacy technician is on a list. The technician receives a registration number upon successful completion of their application. Generally no examination is required for registered technicians. For example, Nevada's board of pharmacy requires approximately the same things as Utah, except for the Laws and Rules examination.

Reciprocity

Reciprocity is the mutual exchange of privileges. This term was first used in pharmacy when dealing with pharmacist licenses. The respective boards of pharmacy developed guidelines to grant licensure to a pharmacist from another state when moving or traveling for work. The idea behind the guidelines was that if a pharmacist had a license in one state, it would be easier to acquire one in another state. There are some pharmacists who have a license in almost all 50 states.

With the advancement of pharmacy technicians, this idea has made its way into technician licensing as well. In many states, one of the potential requirements may be to have a license from another state and proof of a certain amount of hours of work experience. That is then sufficient to receive a license in another state.

National Certification

Certification is when an organization confers recognition to an individual. This recognition is of a higher level of knowledge or practice as a pharmacy technician. In order to gain certification, certain minimum qualifications must be met, a high-level examination must be passed, and a fee paid. Certification also must be renewed in order to remain certified. A pharmacy technician who achieves certification is able to add the designation **CPhT** at the end of their name, which stands for **Certified Pharmacy Technician**. This is much the same as when nurses put RN at the end of their name.

What is interesting is that national certification was originally designed as a higher level of achievement for technicians *already* working in the field. Due to increased demand for well-trained technicians, this has in many cases evolved into a prerequisite for employment rather than an optional feature.

Two organizations are recognized as being able to confer national technician certification—the Pharmacy Technician Certification Board (PTCB) and the National Healthcareer Association (NHA). The names of the exams given by each are the Pharmacy Technician Certification Exam (PTCE), and the Exam for Certified Pharmacy Technicians (ExCPT), respectively.

More information on requirements to take either exam, including cost, testing criteria, pass requirements, and content, can be found at each organization's website. Registering for an exam is done on these websites as well. The question is often which test to take. PTCB was the first and most well-known organization for national certification of technicians, but both exams are generally recognized in most states. It is recommended that students or technicians looking to take an exam research the benefits, cost, and so on for both, as well as ask other technicians or pharmacists which they recommend.

Exam Preparation

There are many books devoted to the subject of national certification preparation. All of them cover the material that is tested on, and most have accompanying CDs with practice tests, flash cards, and the like. Note that most vocational training programs cover a majority of the content from the national exam within their curriculum. In that case, prep books are similar to a Cliff's Notes version of the various textbooks used in school. This is actually good for refreshing on a broad range of material without feeling overwhelmed. There are also websites that have aids for getting ready to take the national exam, including practice tests.

One approach is to take several practice exams to become familiar with the material covered in the national exam. If the score on the practice tests is consistently well above the required passing score, then it would be wise to sign up and take the test. If the score is close to the passing score or below, identification of problem areas is the next step. By working on any areas of difficulty, such as math or drug words, one knows where to focus their efforts. Studying every chapter of every book learned in school is not the most efficient method of preparing for the national certification.

RENEWALS AND CONTINUING EDUCATION

Every state that regulates technicians requires the renewal of licensure in order to continue to work in that state. This renewal typically needs to occur every 2 years, and requires a renewal fee and proof of the completion of continuing education.

Continuing Education Overview

Continuing education (CE) consists of short seminars or courses of instruction in pharmacy practice. Boards of pharmacy require the completion of CEs for renewal to ensure that a technician stays up-to-date on subjects in their scope of practice. The subjects of different CEs can cover areas such as laws and regulations, new developments in pharmacy practice, or even specific drug uses and dosing.

CEs are measured in contact hours, also called credit hours or units. For example, a particular CE could be worth 2.0 contact hours, or 2.0 continuing education units (CEUs). This means that the content of the CE should take approximately 2 hours to learn. Some CEs can be only 1–1.5 hours, and others can count for up to 4 hours of instruction, depending on content.

Every state has its own standards of what constitutes a CE. Some states allow staff meetings to count as a CE, with proper documentation, whereas others require accredited CE credits. The **Accreditation Council for Pharmacy Education (ACPE)** certifies continuing education courses for both pharmacists and pharmacy technicians. A CE course that is accredited will have the ACPE logo on its documentation (Accreditation Council for Pharmacy Education, n.d.).

When a CE is completed, a certificate is issued to the technician. There are several key pieces of information to note, such as the number of contact hours earned, the name of the course, and the course code. These will be important when recording CEs for credit and renewal.

Continuing Education Requirements

Although state requirements vary regarding the number of CEs needed for a technician to renew their license, national certification requires 20 CEUs. This is *not* in addition to the required state amount; CEs can count toward both renewals. For example, if the Nevada Board of Pharmacy requires 12 CEUs, only 8 more would need to be completed in order to meet national certification requirements.

TIPS AND TRICKS
To Renew or Not to Renew?

If a license is allowed to expire, the fines and requirements to reinstate it will vary from state to state, but will ultimately cost more money and effort than keeping licenses current, even if you are not currently working as a pharmacy technician (**Figure 15-1**). You never know when you might need that as a backup means of income, and it is always harder to get back a license than to keep it renewed.

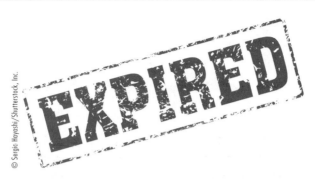

© Sergio Hayashi/Shutterstock, Inc.

FIGURE 15-1 It is wise to keep a license from expiring, even if you are not currently working in the field.

Continuing Education Sources

There are many avenues for obtaining the requisite number of CEs to maintain licensure. These can be found on the Internet, in printed materials, and via live presentations. Even attending a state board of pharmacy meeting can be worth continuing education credit. Some CEs are free, whereas others cost money. A good start would be to conduct a web search for "pharmacy technician continuing education" to investigate possible sources.

IN THE FIELD
NABP CPE Monitor

Following the trend of innovations like the electronic health record (EHR), the National Association of Boards of Pharmacy has developed a central storage program for CE credit for both pharmacists and technicians. This program is known as the NABP CPE Monitor. When a technician completes an ACPE-accredited CE course, this information is transmitted to the CPE Monitor's database. This information can then be accessed by state boards of pharmacy for verification during license renewal.

In order to utilize this database, a technician must sign up to receive an e-profile ID and password by creating a profile. This process does not cost money. Many CE providers ask for this ID so they can submit credit upon completion (National Association of Boards of Pharmacy, n.d.a.).

PROFESSIONAL ORGANIZATIONS

A **professional organization** is a group of practitioners of a particular profession that seek to improve that profession, safeguard the public, and in many cases do both. It does this by advocating guidelines and ethical standards, and providing training. There are many professional organizations in the field of pharmacy. These organizations can be classified in several different ways. Some organizations are strictly for technicians or pharmacists, and some cater to both. There are national organizations and state-specific ones. Another classification can be whether the organization focuses on the community, compounding, or health system setting. Some organizations have been around for 50 years or more, whereas some have only recently been created. And new organizations will continue to form. See **Table 15-1** for a list of the most common national professional organizations that technicians can join.

Table 15-1 Common National Professional Organizations for Pharmacy Technicians

Organization	Web Address
American Association of Pharmacy Technicians (AAPT)	www.pharmacytechnician.com
American Society of Health-System Pharmacists (ASHP)	www.ashp.org
National Pharmacy Technician Association (NPTA)	www.pharmacytechnician.org
Pharmacy Technician Educators Council (PTEC)	www.pharmacytecheducators.com
Society for the Education of Pharmacy Technicians (SEPhT)	www.thesepht.org

Benefits of Membership

Becoming a member of a professional organization is optional for a technician, and not a requirement for employment. In fact, many technicians hold no organizational affiliations. This is, therefore, an excellent area to explore for professional development. There are several very useful benefits to consider. Most, if not all, professional pharmacy organizations provide the following benefits to their members:

- *Continuing education:* Provided online, sent in the mail, or in a newsletter, continuing education is essential for pharmacy technicians to maintain licensure.
- *Current events:* Organizations strive to keep their members abreast of current trends in the field, new legislation, and other important information regarding pharmacy practice.
- *Conferences:* Live meetings hosted annually or more often, these events provide live CE credit and the ability to meet with colleagues.

There are other benefits to joining a professional organization. One is the opportunity to network. Conferences gather like-minded technicians from every region that the organization covers, which can be an invaluable source of contacts. Another aspect is distinction. Membership in an organization can be put on a resume, and demonstrates to a potential employer the technician's dedication. If a technician is a member of a professional organization, he or she could be viewed as taking the profession more seriously, because it is a step above just getting licensed.

Although it is not possible to discuss every professional organization, we can highlight one as an example that is very relevant to the content of this text. The **American Society of Health-System Pharmacists (ASHP)** is the largest organization for hospital pharmacy professionals in the world. ASHP has been one of the largest proponents of advancement in technician practice. Every year ASHP hosts its Midyear Clinical Meeting, a convention that features continuing education and speakers from across the country, including keynote speakers such as former president William Jefferson Clinton. These presentations describe innovations in the field, and many discuss new roles that have been created for pharmacy technicians. A measure of the growing importance of the technician can be seen in the fact that the most recent Midyear Meetings have an entire day's worth of educational programming created by and for technicians.

Choosing an Organization

Although becoming a member of a professional organization is voluntary, if you are considering membership as an option, the next step is to choose which one to join. Why not become a member of every group? Although ambitious, this would be like trying to be in every club or sport in high school. It is rather hard to accomplish, and just looks like someone is trying too hard to fit in; however, two or even three memberships are not unreasonable. A technician who is a member of 30 professional organizations would raise eyebrows, however, and not necessarily in a good way.

When selecting a group to join, it truly comes down to which one fits the best. Comparisons should be made among several groups to determine which one stands out to the technician most.

SUMMARY

It is important to understand the credentials needed to practice as a pharmacy technician. It is equally important to know the requirements needed to maintain or improve these credentials. Continuing education is the key to maintaining licensure, registration, or certification.

Professional organizations can add another credential to a technician's profile. Being active in the larger community of pharmacy professionals increases knowledge, builds connections, and demonstrates commitment on the part of the technician.

When considering a technician for employment or advancement, the quality of their credentials plays a factor in the decision. Although some aspects of gaining credentials may be attainable fairly quickly, other aspects will take experience in the field to develop.

REVIEW QUESTIONS

1. Does the state you live in register or license technicians? Is there a fee to acquire the license or registration? How much is this fee?
2. What are the requirements to become licensed in your state?
3. How often must renewal occur?
4. What is your state's requirement for CE credits for renewal?
5. Does your state have a reciprocity option for technicians from other states?

6. How many national certification exams are available to take in the United States? What are their designations?

7. Are there state professional organizations that pharmacy technicians can join? What might be some benefits of being a member of a state organization in addition to or instead of a national one?

8. Compare and contrast the different national technician organizations. Which seems to be the best to join? Why?

9. What are the benefits of attending conventions and conferences?

10. What are some of the major national conferences that technicians can attend?

REFERENCES

Accreditation Council for Pharmacy Education. (n.d.). Retrieved from https://www.acpe-accredit.org

Credential. (n.d.). In OxfordDictrionaries.com. Retrieved from: http://oxforddictionaries.com/us/definition/american_english/credential?q=credentials

National Association of Boards of Pharmacy. (n.d.a.). CPE monitor service. Retrieved from http://www.nabp.net/programs/cpe-monitor/cpe-monitor-service/

National Association of Boards of Pharmacy. (n.d.b.). Retrieved from http://www.nabp.net

Nevada State Board of Pharmacy. (n.d.). Pharmaceutical technician application. Retrieved from http://bop.nv.gov/uploadedFiles/bopnvgov/content/Services/newapps/PT_Application.pdf

CHAPTER 16

Finding Employment

LEARNING OBJECTIVES

Upon completion of this chapter, you will be able to

1. Discuss the concept of networking and its importance to securing employment
2. Recognize common methods of application for employment
3. Understand the importance of an appropriate resume for application submission
4. Give examples of answers to common interview questions
5. Explain references and their use in the application process

KEY TERMS

Applicant tracking system (ATS)

Networking

Optimize

Reference

Resume

Small talk

INTRODUCTION

According to the U.S. Department of Labor, the job outlook for pharmacy technicians is very good. Job growth is expected to increase 32% by 2020 (Bureau of Labor Statistics, 2012). In what has been a somewhat shaky economy, this positive projection of job growth is a welcome ray of sunshine for those seeking employment.

These above-average projections can be attributed to the demographics associated with pharmacy. Elderly patients are the largest percentage of the pharmacy customer base. These patients have more illnesses and require more medication for treatment. With advances in health care, the average lifespan of a person in the United States has increased dramatically. With that increase there is also a proportional increase in the number of prescriptions that have to be filled, as well as the number of patients admitted to a hospital for treatment. This workload increase necessitates a greater number of technicians in the field.

The knowledge that careers in health care are promising is not limited to a select few individuals. As a result, there are potentially many other technician applicants vying for employment. To compete effectively for employment opportunities, it is important to have a solid understanding of the different aspects that can go into finding a job in the field.

NETWORKING

Merriam-Webster's dictionary defines **networking** as "the cultivation of productive relationships for employment or business" (Networking, n.d.). Everyone has the capacity to network effectively. Some people may start with a more natural affinity for it, but with awareness and practice, this very useful tactic can be utilized by a pharmacy technician to obtain more opportunities in their career.

In reference to the definition, the term *cultivation* is of note. Building relationships takes time and effort, much like tending to a garden. If done properly, the yield in terms of potential job opportunity is well worth the effort.

In order to network effectively, two aspects must be examined—the techniques of how to network and who to network with. There are many schools of thought and opinions when it comes to networking, and you are encouraged to seek out more viewpoints and tips on the Web, in magazines, or in other books. The strategies in this chapter are meant to introduce you to the concept of networking and give some basic starting points to explore.

Networking Techniques

There are various methods to cultivate productive relationships with other pharmacy professionals. Some involve face-to-face communication, whereas others involve electronic methods of interaction. Both are areas that you should devote effort to. As an overview, here are two steps that can be followed to start networking: (1) making connections, and (2) maintaining connections.

Making Connections

Relationships are naturally formed when directly communicating with someone for a significant amount of time, such as in a training or classroom setting. The art of networking is put to the test during brief, introductory communications with relative strangers. In either scenario, the tone of this relationship can be positive or negative, and must be considered when engaging in communications.

The ability to make small talk is one that must be developed to facilitate interactions with new connections. **Small talk** is conversation about items that are not controversial or of deep concern to either party. An old saying is never to talk about religion, politics, or money. Ever. These would be considered controversial subjects. "How much do you make?" "Do you believe in God?" and "Who did you vote for?" would be completely inappropriate and would not help in building contacts while networking. In order to form a relationship, it is important to find small things in common. This breaks the ice and allows more professional-oriented discussion to be introduced later.

Ice-breaking questions in general are well suited to laying the foundation for networking. Note the term *questions*. It is necessary to ask questions to get to know someone. This is the basis for forming a connection (**Figure 16-1**). Some common subjects to talk about would include:

- Pets
- Hometown or time living in current city
- Family
- Favorite foods
- Hobbies
- How someone got into the pharmacy field

These areas and others of a similar nature are considered safe and fairly universal. It is hard to offend someone or cause a negative reaction by asking them what their favorite food is. And everyone has a favorite food of some kind, so it would not lead to a dead end in the conversation.

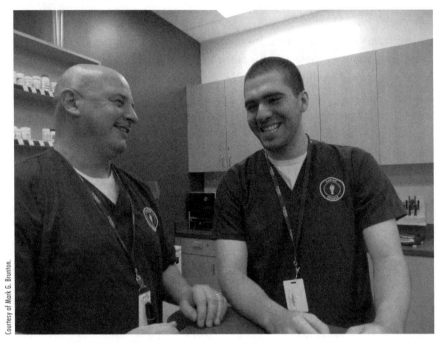

Courtesy of Mark G. Brunton.

FIGURE 16-1 Forming connections via small talk.

TIPS AND TRICKS
The Secret to Making Connections

Many people are not masters of the art of small talk and feel that they do not initiate conversations well. They often feel that they must find things in common to talk about and feel pressure in doing so. The secret to effective small talk is to *let the other person talk*. Being a courteous listener is the secret. In terms of finding things in common, if one does not know much about the subject being discussed, then a good tactic would be to ask for more information. For example, let's say the subject being talked about was hobbies, and the other person says they like to swing dance. A good response would something along the lines of, "I have never done that, but it sounds really interesting. Is it fun?" People generally love talking about their hobbies, and a connection will still be made, even if you do not have experience in that area. The fact that the information was shared forms the connection.

Maintaining Connections

After an initial connection has been made with small talk about common interests, it is time to initiate the next aspect of networking, which can be classified as building relationships. In order to form lasting connections with a colleague, it is necessary to acquire their contact information. This can be an email address, a work phone number, or even an address to send a postcard to. A common way to connect is to ask if the person you are connecting with has a business card. If they do not, then simply ask if they have an email address where you could reach them in the future.

It doesn't do a technician any good to initiate a connection and then never follow up with that connection. That would be the same as planting a seed, but then never watering it. In order to build a connection, it must be kept in contact with. A simple follow-up message is a good start, stating that it was nice to have met the person, and to stay in touch. After that, there should be periodic follow-up communications to maintain that relationship.

Whom to Network With

The answer to this question can be as simple as *everyone* (Doyle, n.d.). This, of course, refers to everyone you meet in the field of pharmacy, whether it is on externship or training, a field trip, or when picking up your own personal prescription from the local retail pharmacy. The saying that almost everyone knows regarding employment is that "it's not what you know, it's who you know." Although true, a better statement would be "it is what you know *and* who you know." The knowledge and training needed to be a technician are necessary, but the connections built with people in the field are an aspect that cannot be ignored. A large percentage of jobs available to a pharmacy technician are never posted and are heard about only through connections (**Figure 16-2**).

Let's examine some of the people that can be connected with for networking purposes.

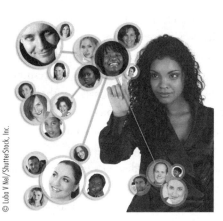

© Luba V Nel/ShutterStock, Inc.

FIGURE 16-2 Networking is a key skill for increased employment opportunities.

- *Classmates:* If you are in a classroom setting, look around you. Every technician student in that class has the potential to either hear of a job they can tell you about or actually be in a position to hire you at some point in the future. With that perspective in mind, it would be prudent to maintain positive relationships with fellow technician trainees, and work at building connections with them. This is the first chance many will get to begin networking, and is good practice.

- *Training preceptors and staff:* When gaining practical experience in a hospital pharmacy setting, all of the pharmacy staff are a potential network. Often when training, a site may not be hiring at that particular time. This is when a technician trainee might lose motivation and enthusiasm. It does not mean that this site will not hire a week or a month from that point, however, and they will call the trainee who made the best impression. If a training site is impressed enough with the performance of a student, they have also been known to recommend them to other facilities that are hiring, even if they are not.

APPLYING FOR A POSITION

Finding job opportunities and applying for them can be one of the most challenging and stressful times of a technician's career. It is a time of uncertainty, and can feel like searching for a needle in a haystack. Understanding some of the common methods used and items needed during this process can help shed some light on the subject.

Resumes

A **resume** is the summary of qualifications of an applicant in a given field. It can also be an important part of the application process. A pharmacy technician should always have an up-to-date resume, even if they are already employed. You can find countless formats and suggestions for how to write an effective resume on the Web; this text does not advocate any one type of resume over another. The resume format is a personal choice for the applicant, and should be diverse and unique, as long as it maintains acceptable conventions. There are some points to address that can help guide the creation of this document.

There are many Internet resources available that list elements to review when writing a resume to ensure that errors are not made and nothing is forgotten. Although a resume can be unique to each applicant, the following lists some of the universal elements to be aware of during its creation:

- Font type and size should be consistent and easily read either digitally or in print form.

- The spacing between different areas of the resume should be consistent; use white space effectively.
- Use spell and grammar check, and then have someone you know review it. It is a wise decision to have an instructor or other pharmacy professional that you have networked with be the second or even third set of eyes to look at your resume. They can offer extremely useful suggestions for content, and not all spelling errors are caught by automated programs.
- Are all personal contact information items current? Nothing is worse than not getting a call for an interview because an old phone number was on the resume.

There should be at least two versions of a resume on hand when needed. One version can utilize whatever formatting or design elements the applicant prefers, and would be used for physical submission to a prospective employer. The other version should have no formatting whatsoever. The content should be the same, but without any unique fonts, borders, or the like. This version would be used for online submissions, which will be discussed in the next section of this chapter.

TIPS AND TRICKS
Resume Resurrection

After working at one place for a while, the need for a resume diminishes. If you should suddenly need one again, due to a layoff or new job opportunity, for example, many times a technician has to scramble and search for their old resume. It is often necessary to have to start from scratch. An effective solution to this problem is to store your resume on the Web. A simple way to do this is to email it as an attachment to yourself and save the email. Other options include using cloud-based storage solutions. This ensures that no matter where or when, as long as you have access to the Internet, you have access to your resume.

Online Applications

Most health systems use an online application process to employ pharmacy technicians (**Figure 16-3**). This system takes the place of traditional paper applications that are filled out by hand, and in some ways is very similar. Due to the

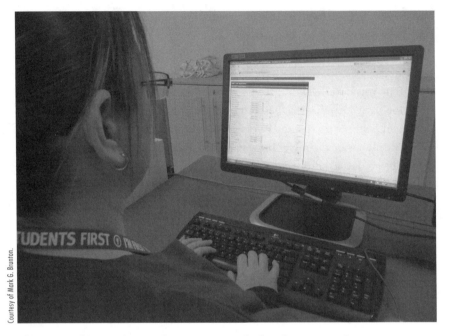

FIGURE 16-3 Online applications are used often for many technician positions.

nature of online applications, there are more options and capabilities to be aware of than with older application processes.

Career hunting websites such as Monster.com and Career Builder are middle-men, in terms of application submission. An alternative is to find the website of the health systems in your region and locate the section of their site for employment opportunities. Note that many hospitals are part of a larger company that may encompass several facilities, and there may be one primary website for all of them.

To apply for posted positions with a particular company, it is usually necessary to register a profile with their system. This profile includes basic information such as name and address, an uploaded resume, and completion of their online application form. Once that has been completed, an applicant can submit for a posted position.

Online Optimization

To **optimize** something is to make it as effective as possible. In the case of online applications, this is especially important. Many systems use what is known as an **applicant tracking system (ATS)** (Salpeter, 2012). This is specialized software that screens applications and sorts them based on keywords or phrases that it identifies in each particular application. This screening software saves the employer from having to review every application submitted. This also means that a live employer might not actually review *your* application if it doesn't rate as high on the ATS as another application.

Optimizing an application makes it as effective as it can be when encountering this type of screening process. In order to optimize an application, it and the attached resume should be reviewed in comparison to the position being applied for. The job description is a roadmap for identifying what the employer is looking for in a candidate. Using the same jargon, terms, and industry-specific buzzwords as the job description increases the attractiveness of the application to the ATS software. For example, if a position's job description deals with IV compounding, the applicant should make sure that "sterile compounding," "aseptic technique," and other related terms are in their application for that position.

It is important to remember that new postings on company websites can pop up at any time, and just because an application was submitted in response to one posting, it is not automatically reposted for every position. That action must be performed by the applicant for each individual posting.

TIPS AND TRICKS
Bypassing the ATS

Although the ATS is a factor that needs to be considered when applying online, it is not necessarily the only gatekeeper to getting called for an interview. If a networking connection has been made with a supervisor in that particular pharmacy, they can often request that a particular candidate's resume or application get pushed through to them for review, regardless of the ATS screening process. In order to achieve this, it is important to notify that contact when submitting an application for a position so they can be on the lookout for it.

INTERVIEWING

Interviewing is another area that many people are not comfortable with, and which can cause high levels of stress and fear during the application process. It is unfortunately a necessary step in the process to gain employment. Many no-

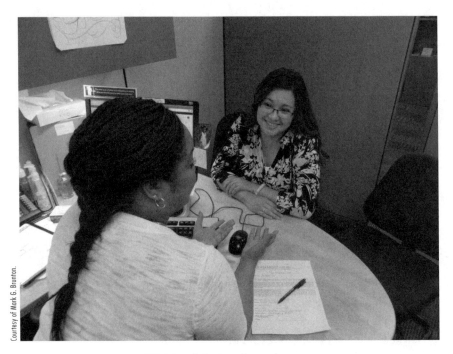

FIGURE 16-4 A traditional interview.

doubt-qualified technicians do not get hired because of a botched interview. Proper behavior and tactics can be learned, however, to combat this (**Figure 16-4**). Awareness of the outline of an interview can help to control involuntary stress.

Appearance and Punctuality

These two areas cannot be stressed enough. An applicant could answer every interview question perfectly, have a great attitude, and still not get hired if appearance and punctuality are not up to the employer's standards. Business casual attire is recommended for best results in terms of appearance. Almost all resources available on the subject of punctuality suggest arriving at the interview at least 30 minutes early. This creates a buffer for any unexpected delays or circumstances, such as traffic, getting lost, or the like. It is much better to have time to spare than be late. Being late to an interview conveys a lack of respect for the interviewer's time.

Mindset and Perspective

There are many potential questions a hiring manager could ask, and many suggested answers to the most common ones. These lists of interview questions are widely available, and you are encouraged to review them. The suggested answers should not be memorized, however, because the response will seem fake when delivered. The best strategy is to analyze the content of the responses and find a way to put it into your own words. This will ensure that responses feel genuine when given.

The most important concept to keep in mind is that an interview is not as scary as many make it out to be. An interview is nothing more than a chance for an employer to *get to know you*, and more importantly, get to know whether you are someone they can see working on their team. Although you want to present your best first impression, make it an honest impression. Do not try to be someone or something that you are not.

Interviewers will ask questions related to their practice setting. As with an application, it is good to be able to speak the jargon and use appropriate terminology when discussing your qualifications. In a health system setting, being able to discuss your competency with sterile product preparation and automation will go a long way toward demonstrating your ability to function in their work setting.

TIPS AND TRICKS
The Guided Tour Interview

A tactic sometimes used by interviewers in the field is to give a tour of the department during the interview. This is useful to both the applicant and the hiring supervisor. By giving an overview of the department, a hiring supervisor can gauge an applicant's ability to handle the requirements of the position. It is useful to the applicant in that it may answer questions about what they will be expected to do if hired, and gives them a sense of the feel of the department. There are some notes to be aware of in this type of interview:

- *Introductions:* Often the hiring supervisor will introduce an applicant to other employees in the pharmacy. Treat these interactions the same as you would the introduction to the supervisor. Be courteous and friendly. The supervisor will ask staff about their impressions of the applicant when making the final hiring decision.
- *Sense of security:* If the applicant has been trying to convey a false impression, this is the time when that pretense tends to slip. Be consistent in behavior. By being honest and genuine in an interview, this is a nonissue.

- *Assess the department:* Besides learning the general operations of the pharmacy, this is a chance for an applicant to get a feel for the department. Are the employees happy? Do pharmacists or technicians seem grouchy or stressed out? This can alert the applicant to decide whether they actually want to take a position in a given setting.

By being aware of the elements of a guided tour scenario, an applying technician can navigate this type of interview just as successfully as a traditional sit-down one.

TIPS AND TRICKS
The Power of Silence

Silence is sometimes considered a dirty tactic to be used by an interviewer, but it is nonetheless an effective one. An interviewer using this technique allows silence to stretch during an interview, usually after asking a question. After an applicant has responded to the question, the interviewer will remain silent, as if to invite the applicant to add more. Usually an applicant will find the silence uncomfortable, and will continue to talk, which can potentially reveal more than the applicant intended in the interview.

By understanding the tactic, you can counter it. A simple method is to ask the interviewer if they would like to know more, or what else you can elaborate on. This then requires the interviewer to respond, which breaks the uncomfortable silence and helps to progress the interview.

Follow Up

With numerous candidates for a position, it is both polite and useful to follow up with a thank you message after the interview. This can be in the form of a mailed card or an email message, and is usually sent 1–2 days after an interview. A thank you note conveys how much you appreciated the interviewer's time and helps keep your name in their considerations for employment.

REFERENCES

A professional **reference** is a person who can vouch for your qualifications as a pharmacy technician. Your references should be drawn from your professional network described previously. It is customary to ask a person if they would be a reference for you. Understand that in order to have good references, it is important to make a good impression on them, so that they have good things to say about you. Consider that a reference's reputation is potentially at stake when recommending someone for employment. Keep that in mind when building your network to ensure that a colleague or supervisor will *want* to be your reference in the future. When first starting your career as a pharmacy technician, here are some potential sources for references:

- *Instructors and program chairs:* These individuals can speak to a student's performance while in school, grade point average, punctuality, and demeanor, as well as general competency.
- *Training site personnel:* Preceptors, pharmacists, pharmacy directors, and other technicians encountered during clinical training are also invaluable sources for references.

These individuals are able to give excellent critiques of your qualifications, because they are knowledgeable about the field being entered. Family members and friends generally are not considered professional references and should not be used. Classmates are a secondary option. After working in the field, past supervisors and coworkers become viable references as well.

It is a good practice to remind or alert a reference when using them on an application, even if they have already given their consent in the past. This is to let them know that they may be receiving a call about your qualifications. It also allows them time to think about how best to describe you, so they are not caught off guard. This gives the reference a chance to represent you with the best possible description.

SUMMARY

Many elements go into a successful job search and securing employment. By building a strong network of professionals in the field, even more opportunities for employment become available. An up-to-date resume that is optimized helps increase the chances of being called in for an interview. Knowing the structure of the online application process is critical to actually applying for a position in the current job market. Maintaining an honest and relaxed yet professional demeanor in an interview will lead to more job offers. Having a solid list of available references can be the tipping point to receiving the call to work for a given employer.

REVIEW QUESTIONS

1. Name three people you could practice making connections with. How would you develop this skill personally?
2. What are some of the benefits of networking?
3. Name three locations where you could make legitimate connections with pharmacy professionals.
4. Define *optimization*. What are some areas that can benefit from this concept in addition to online applications?
5. What are some keywords that would be useful to put in an online application for a health system position in regards to an ATS?
6. Research common interview questions. Which ones do you think a hiring manager for a pharmacy might ask?
7. What are some effective answers to the questions found for the previous question?
8. Besides the traditional sit-down and guided tour interviews, are there other types of interviews that may be encountered? Would your strategy change? Why or why not?
9. What would be a good way to ask someone to be a reference?
10. Who would make a good reference in the field of pharmacy?

REFERENCES

Bureau of Labor Statistics. (2012). Occupational outlook handbook: Pharmacy technicians. Retrieved from http://www.bls.gov/ooh/healthcare/pharmacy-technicians.htm

Doyle, A. (n.d.). Job search and career networking tips: The importance of career networking. Retrieved from http://jobsearch.about.com/od/networking/a/networkingtips.htm

Networking. (n.d.). In Merriam-Webster.com. Retrieved from http://www.merriam-webster.com/dictionary/networking

Salpeter, M. (2012, July 11). The 9 best tips for submitting an online job application. Retrieved from http://money.usnews.com/money/blogs/outside-voices-careers/2012/07/11/the-9-best-tips-for-submitting-an-online-job-application

Glossary

Accountability—An obligation or willingness to accept responsibility for one's actions.

Accreditation Council for Pharmacy Education (ACPE)—An organization that approves the content of continuing education programs.

Active listening—A technique in which the listener repeats back the information communicated to them by the sender.

Admissions—Refers to a patient when admitted to hospital, as well as necessary demographic information.

Admissions, discharges, and transfers (ADT) system—A common abbreviation used to define a hospital's software program that deals with patient information regarding admissions, discharges, and transfers.

Adverse drug event (ADE)—Any injury resulting from the use of a drug.

Adverse drug reaction (ADR)—A response to a drug that is noxious and unintended, and that occurs at normal doses for said drug.

American Society of Health-System Pharmacists (ASHP)—A national professional organization that works on behalf of pharmacists and pharmacy technicians who practice in hospitals and health systems.

Ampule—Glass container with no rubber stopper used for IV medications.

Appearance—The outward or visible aspect of a person.

Applicant tracking system—Specialized software that screens applications and sorts them based on keywords or phrases.

Aseptic technique—Procedures used when compounding IV preparations in order to prevent contamination of the product.

Attitude—A way of thinking or feeling that is usually reflected in a person's behavior.

Automated dispensing cabinet (ADC)—Device used to dispense medication to nurses in the nursing unit, similar to a bank ATM.

Automation—The use of technology to make tasks easier.

Biometrics—Technology that analyzes unique biological characteristics for identity verification.

Blind count—Setting used for controlled substances or high-cost medications that requires a manual inventory count by a user when accessing in an automated dispensing cabinet.

Board of pharmacy—Organization that handles the regulatory requirements for pharmacy in a given state.

Budget—A limited supply of something.

Bulk—Bottle of pills or capsules, typically in quantities of 30, 50, 100, 1,000, and so forth.

Business casual—A style of clothing worn by businesspeople at work that is slightly more casual than traditional formal work attire.

Calibration—Comparing a device's stated measurement against another scale of measure to determine accuracy.

Central supply—Department that provides the hospital with all consumable products used that are not medications, including bandages, syringes, toiletries, and the like.

Certification—When an organization confers recognition to an individual.

Certified Pharmacy Technician (CPhT)—A title granted to pharmacy technicians who pass a national certification examination.

Chain of command—The line of authority and responsibility along which orders are passed.

Closed system transfer device (CSTD)—A generic term for any device that connects a vial of medication with the fluid it will be mixed in, without actually mixing them.

Code cart—A portable storage unit of all medications and devices that could potentially be needed during a code event.

Communication—The process of delivering a message.

Compounded sterile preparations (CSPs)—Term for IV preparations, but can also encompass certain other medications, such as topical eye preparations or other substances that need to be made in a sterile environment.

Compounding—Mixing substances.

Computer on wheels (COW)—A portable computer workstation used by nurses.

Computerized physician order entry (CPOE)—Allows a doctor to input their orders for a patient directly into the hospital computer system.

Concentration—The amount of drug in a given volume of solution.

Connectivity—The ability of different computer systems and devices to communicate with one another.

Continuing education (CE)—Short seminars or courses of instruction in pharmacy practice, required for renewal of licensure.

Coring—When a piece of the rubber stopper is separated from a vial and falls into the solution.

Credentials—A qualification, achievement, personal quality, or the like, used to indicate suitability for something.

Critical override—A setting for automated dispensing cabinets where all medications can be overridden.

Critical site—Any area where direct contact with the medication or IV solution occurs.

Critical thinking—The mental process of actively and skillfully conceptualizing, applying, analyzing, synthesizing, and evaluating information to reach an answer or conclusion.

DEA 222 form—A legal document required by the Drug Enforcement Administration to place orders for class II medications.

Decentralized pharmacy—Composed of a main pharmacy and several smaller pharmacies located throughout a facility.

Decorum—Element of etiquette that describes the appropriate social behavior within a set situation.

Diluent—Any liquid that is used to dissolve a solid into a solution.

Discharge—When patients leave the care of the hospital.

Discrepancy (ADC)—Alert generated when a controlled substance or other monitored drug is unaccounted for in an automated dispensing cabinet.

Discrepancy (narcotic log book)—An error between the narcotic log and the physical inventory of a medication.

Diversion—Term used for theft in the pharmacy.

Dose cup—Unit dose containers that can hold volumes from 5 ml to 45 ml, as necessary, for different types of medications.

Dress code—The rules for appropriate attire in a given facility.

Electronic health record (EHR)—A patient's medical record of care, shared among all healthcare providers electronically.

Electronic medication administration record (EMAR)—Documents when medication is given to a patient by nursing.

Entitlement—A claim to something.

Fast movers—Certain medications that are used heavily in a given facility.

Fight or flight—The body's natural reaction to stressful situations.

First air—The object that first comes into contact with air from a HEPA filter.

Food and Drug Administration Adverse Event Reporting System (FAERS)—A database that contains information on adverse event and medication error reports submitted to the Food and Drug Administration.

Formulary—List of all medications approved for use in a given facility.

Gauge—A measurement of how wide the diameter is of the interior portion of a needle.

Grooming—To care for one's appearance.

Health system—Term for what has traditionally been known as a hospital setting.

High efficiency particulate air (HEPA)—A type of filter that produces ultra-clean air while compounding sterile products.

Hospital information system (HIS)—Umbrella term for all computer programs and systems used in a hospital setting.

Humbleness—A modest opinion or estimate of one's own importance, rank, and so on.

Institute for Safe Medication Practices (ISMP)—A nonprofit entity dedicated to medication safety improvement.

Inventory—The actual number of medications on hand in a given automated dispensing cabinet or in the entire hospital.

Lyophilized—Freeze-dried medication.

Medication error—Any preventable event that may cause or lead to inappropriate medication use or patient harm while the medication is in the control of the healthcare professional, patient, or consumer.

Medication misadventure—Term used by pharmacy for many medication errors and categories.

Medication reconciliation—The process of comparing a patient's medication orders to all of the medications that the patient has been taking prior to admission to a hospital.

Medmarx—A program that documents medication errors electronically within a given facility.

MedWatch—A program run by the Food and Drug Administration to inform both healthcare practitioners and the general public about safety concerns regarding medications.

Mindset—A fixed mental attitude or disposition that predetermines a person's responses to and interpretations of situations.

Multiple dose vial (MDV)—Vial intended for multiple uses; contains preservatives.

Narcotic log book—Written method of keeping inventory of controlled substances.

National Association of Boards of Pharmacy (NABP)—Organization that assists state boards of pharmacy in developing, implementing, and enforcing uniform standards relating to pharmacies. Also manages the CE Monitor program.

National Coordinating Council for Medication Error Reporting and Prevention (NCC MERP)—Created at the request of the U.S. Pharmacopeia; made up of several national organizations.

Networking—The cultivation of productive relationships for employment or business.

Nonverbal communication—The actions of both the sender and receiver during communication that do not involve words.

Optimize—To make as effective as possible.

Oral syringe—A syringe used for administering oral liquid medication to a patient.

Order set—A programmed list of medications that can be selected during order entry.

Override—When a medication is removed from an automated dispensing cabinet prior to the order for the medication being reviewed and approved by a pharmacist.

Par level—The minimum and maximum amount of a drug that should be loaded into a given machine.

Pass-through—A chamber for moving items into and out of a barrier isolator.

Pathogen—Disease-causing agents, such as bacteria, fungi, and viruses.

Patient ID—A unique number assigned to a patient for the duration of their visit.

Patient lookup—Allows one to select a specific patient from the pharmacy software database.

Patient profile—Record of a specific patient in the facility.

Perception—The recognition or appreciation of moral, psychological, or aesthetic qualities.

Professional organization—A group of practitioners of a particular profession that seek to improve that profession, safeguard the public, and in many cases both.

Punctuality—The strict observance of an appointed or regular time.

Recall—When a specific lot of medication is asked to be returned to the manufacturer.

Receiver—The person who is interpreting a message during communication.

Reciprocity—The mutual exchange of privileges.

Reconstitution—The process of adding a diluent to a lyophilized powder to turn it into a solution.

Reference—A person who can vouch for your qualifications.

Repackaging—Transferring a medication from a bulk container to a unit dose container.

Repackaging control log—A record of repackaging procedure and ingredient information.

Resume—A summary of qualifications of an applicant in a given field.

Satellite pharmacy—Smaller pharmacies located throughout a hospital as part of the decentralized model.

Scheduled drug—A controlled substance or a drug that has the potential for abuse.

Scrubs—Lightweight garments that were originally designed as sterile garb for use in an operating room.

Sender—The person who is conveying information during communication.

Sentinel event—Joint Commission term for an unexpected occurrence involving death or serious physical or psychological injury, or the risk thereof.

Sig—Short for *signa*, a Latin term used in prescription writing when referring to directions for the patient.

Sig codes—Programmed abbreviations for common sig instructions for order entry operations.

Single dose vial (SDV)—Vial intended for a single use; does not have preservatives.

Small talk—Conversation about items that are not controversial or of deep concern to either party.

Spike—A short, very large plastic needle.

Standard stock—A group of medications that should never be unloaded from a station, regardless of whether a patient currently has an order for them.

Standardized order set—A printed set of orders for procedures or medications commonly done in a given setting.

Sterile—Free from germs or microorganisms.

Stock outs—When a medication is completely empty in a given automated dispensing cabinet.

Stress—The physical and mental reaction to threatening situations.

Syringe—The primary device used to withdraw medication from a vial or ampule and transfer it to an IV solution.

Tall man letters—Letters within printed drug names that are in capitals in order to highlight differences between similar looking medication names to the reader.

The Joint Commission (TJC)—Nonprofit organization that evaluates hospitals' adherence to minimum standards of patient care.

Tone—The pitch and inflection used when speaking.

Total parenteral nutrition (TPN)—A very specialized form of IV preparation that provides all of the nutritional needs for a patient via the IV route.

Transfer—Occurs when a patient is moved from one location to another within the facility.

Trigger word—A word that immediately causes a certain emotional reaction in a listener.

Troubleshooting—A systematic approach to solving problems quickly and efficiently.

Turnaround time—How long it takes from the point an order has been written until the medication is administered to the patient.

Unit dose—A single dose of medication packaged for individual use.

United States Pharmacopeia (USP)—A compendium of standards for medication, food, and dietary supplements for the entire nation.

Verbal communication—The words used to communicate a message to a recipient.

Vial—A glass container with a rubber stopper over the opening used for IV medications.

Want list—A document in which pharmacy staff can write down items for the buyer to order.

Warning screens—Pop-up windows in a computer program that activate when certain criteria are met when entering orders.

Index

Note: Page numbers followed by *b, f,* or *t* indicate material in boxes, figures, or tables, respectively.